Craft Weed

Craft Weed

Family Farming and the Future of the Marijuana Industry

Ryan Stoa

The MIT Press
Cambridge, Massachusetts
London, England

This book was set in Stone Serif by Westchester Publishing Services. Printed and bound in the United States of America.

Library of Congress Cataloging-in-Publication Data

Names: Stoa, Ryan, author.
Title: Craft weed : family farming and the future of the marijuana industry / Ryan Stoa.
Description: Cambridge, MA ; London, England : The MIT Press, [2018] |
    Includes bibliographical references and index.
Identifiers: LCCN 2018010203 | ISBN 9780262038867 (hardcover : alk. paper)
Subjects: LCSH: Cannabis--United States. | Marijuana industry--United States.
Classification: LCC SB295.C35 S742 2018 | DDC 633.7/90973--dc23
    LC record available at https://lccn.loc.gov/2018010203

10 9 8 7 6 5 4 3 2 1

For John

Contents

Acknowledgments

Many people empowered and inspired me to write this book. My thanks first to the many farmers and marijuana industry stakeholders who agreed to speak with me, share their stories, and welcome me into their community. This book would not have been possible without their insight and acceptance.

My research on marijuana agriculture has been supported by a multitude of institutions and publications that enabled, sharpened, and disseminated my work, including the Concordia University School of Law, Florida International University College of Law, *Harvard Law and Policy Review*, *Florida Law Review*, *Hastings Law Journal*, and *McGeorge Law Review*. Bartholomew Stoddard and Adam Rodriguez provided thorough and timely research assistance, and were instrumental contributors.

I am grateful to my editor, Beth Clevenger, for sharing my vision for this book and bringing it to life. Her care and enthusiasm for this project surpassed my expectations.

It is unlikely that I can fully grasp the extent to which my parents made this book possible. At the very least, I can say that their editorial judgments on the manuscript made this a much better book. *Merci*.

Finally, to John, my brother and my best friend, for whom my deepest gratitude is insufficient. I would be lost without his wisdom, generosity, and encouragement.

Boise, Idaho
June 2018

1 The Myth of Big Marijuana

Farming looks mighty easy when your plow is a pencil, and you're a thousand miles from the corn field.

—Dwight Eisenhower, thirty-fourth president of the United States

The first time I stepped foot on a marijuana farm, I couldn't see a thing. It was late at night, and it had taken me almost twenty-four hours to get there from Miami, Florida. I had been working on an article about the water rights of marijuana farmers for the past few months, but since most of these farmers aren't in the habit of discussing their personal matters online or over the phone, I decided to get on a plane to San Francisco and go straight to the source. My destination was in Humboldt County, one of three counties in northern California that make up the "Emerald Triangle," the agricultural heart and soul of the marijuana industry.

When my eyes adjusted to the darkness, my host, Jack, led me to the cabin where I'd be staying. But the cabin was no ordinary cabin. An adjacent room was filled with oak barrels holding Syrah and Cabernet, and a veranda looked out onto several acres of vineyard. "That's unusual," I thought to myself. Touring the farm the next day, Jack showed me his marijuana plants. They were growing vigorously under the California sun, organized in neat rows and labeled with identifying notes. The operation was all very professional, with precise methods for watering, nurturing, and harvesting the plants. Timing was of the essence, Jack told me. Fall out of step with the sun's rhythms, and a crop's growth cycle would be disrupted. Though northern California was a hotbed of marijuana cultivation, Jack's business was thriving because of a meticulous attention to detail. His marijuana fetched prices that reflected a quality product.

Jack is a viticulturist, winemaker, forest manager, and marijuana farmer, among other trades. He is a student of agriculture, having apprenticed with Cuban tobacco farmers, Senegalese goat herders, and French vintners when he was in his early twenties. When his education took him to the Emerald Triangle, he knew he had found his calling. Jack has a knack for growing plants, and perhaps more importantly, for cultivating the human relationships that businesses need to survive. Both are vital traits for a marijuana farmer in these legally ambiguous times.

One of the relationships Jack cultivates is the one he has with me. In addition to being my host, Jack is also my friend—we've known each other since before I can remember. Knowing him, I wasn't surprised to see him engaged in all manner of small-scale agriculture. But when he introduced me to other farmers in the region, the story was much the same; the farmers were passionate about their craft, though in many cases marijuana wasn't the only crop under cultivation. In addition to grapes, farmers grew and marketed seasonal fruits, vegetables, and flowers. Many raised chickens and honey bees, or stocked fish in nearby ponds. Theirs is a homesteading lifestyle, and the remote, isolated nature of marijuana farming requires a diverse skill set. You don't have to go far to find skilled carpenters, cooks, or musicians. A laborer might harvest marijuana one week, and guide rafting trips the next. It is an intimate and tight-knit community, where one person can be a friend, a tenant, and an employee all at the same time. These days, the local police are fond of saying that raids are "complaint-driven." True or not, farming communities seem to believe the mantra, and take every measure to maintain the peace.

Some of the older generation of farmers have been in Humboldt County for decades, and they bring wisdom and institutional memory to the region. Many settled in northern California during the back-to-the-land movement of the 1960s, when progressives fled their city lives in exchange for a more rural, ecologically connected existence. Others came as mining or timber workers, found paradise, and never left. Today many farmers are young and ambitious "ganjapreneurs," but the ethics of the older generation are still reflected in the community's reverence for self-reliance and sustainability.

Jack made sure I was introduced to an older couple who had been hosting open-to-anyone "Sunday Waffles" parties every week for over four decades. He was anxious for me to try their fifty-year-old sourdough culture, hoping it would be as delightful a culinary experience for me as it is for him (it was). Other comically wholesome events in the community include Wednesday afternoon barbeques at the fire station, twice-weekly volleyball games, and a community potluck every third Thursday. I attended as many of these gatherings as I could, and as Jack's guest I was welcomed with open arms. After all was said and done, my first visit to Humboldt County left me with an idyllic image of the modern-day marijuana farming community.

Needless to say, these scenes ran counter to my expectations. My research on marijuana farms to that point had consisted largely of the descriptions contained in news reports of police raids. Typically, those farms were either trespass grows (short-term, large-scale operations on public lands, a method used to reduce one's exposure and liability) or bare-bones private grows with transient tenants. In both cases, the scene was similar. Land gets cleared, makeshift irrigation schemes suck water from nearby streams, trash and propane canisters are strewn about haphazardly, and all types of fertilizers and pesticides are used to maximize yields as quickly as possible.

The marijuana farmers I met painted a decidedly different picture. Theirs is a farming community in tune with itself, the land, and the industry it wants to be a part of. Farmers owned their own land, took care of a familiar crew of workers, and complied with local regulations (to the extent there are any). The marijuana farmers I met were engaged in the kind of local, sustainable, high-quality, small-scale agriculture that the modern food movement likes to put on a pedestal. Cultivating marijuana had revitalized the idea of the American family farm.

At least in this remote corner of the country it had. Elsewhere, the prospects for marijuana agriculture were less rosy. Colorado's nascent marijuana industry—state-legal since 2012—was struggling to navigate a farming culture that assumed cultivation should take place indoors, in large warehouses, where conditions can be controlled but energy costs are sky-high. In Ohio, marijuana legalization advocates were forced to lobby *against* a legalization initiative in 2015. The measure would have granted exclusive farming rights to a select few well-connected companies. Not surprisingly, the proposed oligopoly didn't sit well with the majority of Ohio voters.

Lately, though, the doom and gloom has taken on a big-picture perspective. The prospect of widespread (and perhaps someday federal) legalization has given rise to a fear that corporations will take over the marijuana industry. According to this narrative, a few large farms will flood the market with cheap, generic marijuana, running small-scale farmers out of business.

Marijuana will become an agricultural commodity, and the free market will eventually lead to market consolidation. I like to call this the Big Marijuana prophecy, and you don't have to look very far to find it.

In May 2013, only six months after Washington State legalized recreational marijuana, a tech entrepreneur named Jamen Shively held a press conference in Seattle. The room was buzzing with reporters, cameras, and jostling entrepreneurs. They had all come to hear what Shively had promised would be a game-changing announcement. "We are Big Marijuana," he said. "We are moving forward with plans to build a national and eventually international network of cannabis businesses. We are going to mint more millionaires than Microsoft."[1] Shively was accompanied by Vicente Fox, the former president of Mexico. Fox touted the plan's potential to end the war on drugs, and the message coming out of the event—The Era of Big Marijuana Is upon Us— made an easy headline for media outlets around the country.

Shively was educated at Berkeley and MIT, but his background doesn't reveal any meaningful experience with the marijuana industry—before a stint with Microsoft, Shively worked with tech start-ups, cement companies, and cybercafés.[2] His plan didn't appear to be on solid legal ground, either. Licensing a global network of marijuana businesses would run afoul of national and international drug laws, a detail Shively hadn't yet accounted for. "I don't know how exactly that would be done, but I know it's been done in other industries," he offered.[3] Before long, his business would run into one stumbling block after another. Nonetheless, some wondered if Shively would become the "Bill Gates of Weed." Despite the questionable merits of his proposal, Shively became a media sensation, and investors followed. It seemed he had tapped into a growing public sentiment that, sooner or later, the counterculture marijuana industry would be taken over by corporate interests.

Shively was by no means the only one to feed into the Big Marijuana prophecy. The CEO of another high-profile marijuana firm echoed the familiar rhetoric: "We see the inevitability of large, well-run companies to sell cannabis. That train left the station a long time ago."[4] Derek Peterson, CEO of Terra Tech, a marijuana supply company, echoed those thoughts: "We're a mass-produced society, from the food we eat to the television we watch. Ultimately, big alcohol or big tobacco is going to come into this space. I just can't imagine that won't happen."[5]

It's not surprising that marijuana entrepreneurs are peddling the Big Marijuana narrative. After all, they need investors to buy into the hype. But even neutral observers see the rise of Big Marijuana as likely, if foreboding. In a 2014 study, researchers from the University of California, San Francisco, poured through decades of previously confidential internal communications of tobacco company strategists and executives. They found evidence that, as far back as the 1970s, tobacco companies were looking into marijuana as a potential or rival product. A few corporate documents were all they needed to see to conclude that "legalizing marijuana opens the market to major corporations, including tobacco companies, which have the financial resources, product design technology…, marketing muscle, and political clout to transform the marijuana market."[6] As a result, the authors urged regulators to prevent big companies from taking over the marijuana market and causing a "public health epidemic."

Meanwhile, in the traditional marijuana farming regions of northern California, the fear of a Big Marijuana takeover is palpable. In 2010, California voters decisively rejected Proposition 19, a measure that would have legalized recreational marijuana and commercial cultivation. The usual arguments against legalization were made by skeptics who were concerned about marijuana's impact on public health and safety. What came as a surprise to many, however, was an apparent lack of support for legalization from the Emerald Triangle, where local economies are dominated by, and dependent on, marijuana cultivation. Voters there were *less* enthusiastic about marijuana legalization than the state as a whole. In Trinity County, one of the three counties that make up the Emerald Triangle (besides Humboldt, the other is Mendocino), the measure barely received 40 percent support.

The simple narrative that emerged to explain the Emerald Triangle vote was that marijuana farmers were being driven by greed. The price of marijuana, after all, is inflated on the black market, and having been successful operating in the shadows for so long, these farmers were perfectly happy to maintain the prohibition status quo. The narrative was misleading but not altogether unfounded. Many opponents of legalization voiced concerns that Proposition 19 was vague and would prove difficult to enforce. Marijuana farmers also feared that the law's ambiguous language would allow Big Marijuana conglomerates to flourish. They sensed that an unregulated environment—or a regulated environment stacked against them—might create more problems than it solved. If marijuana agriculture was left unchecked, large-scale producers would threaten to drive out California's small-scale marijuana farms.

Marijuana agriculture is now a major economic force in states like California and Oregon, and politicians have taken notice of the Big Marijuana prophecy. Gavin Newsom—California's lieutenant governor—is a 2018 gubernatorial candidate and marijuana legalization advocate. He chaired the state's Blue Ribbon Commission on Marijuana Policy, hoping to prepare California for the end of prohibition. Newsom recognizes the Big Marijuana threat. "Legalization should not be about replacing one cartel with another," he said.[7]

In states without a track record of marijuana cultivation, some politicians have used the Big Marijuana prophecy to lobby against legalization in the first place. The Massachusetts governor and attorney general, joined by Boston's mayor, came out against marijuana legalization in 2016. They felt the state was unprepared to reckon with big businesses taking over the industry, and expressed skepticism that Big Marijuana would control the market responsibly. "Motivated by the profit potential of dominating a new marketplace, proponents know it's not in their best interest," they wrote in a *Boston Globe* op-ed.[8] They might well be right.

One thing is clear: if the Big Marijuana prophecy comes true, there won't be a shortage of likely culprits. Big Tobacco and Big Alcohol know how to produce and sell inhalants and intoxicants. Big Agriculture cultivates prodigious quantities of agricultural commodities. Big Pharmaceuticals can realize the medical and commercial potential of psychoactive drugs. And Wall Street and Silicon Valley bring investors and disruptive technologies.

Marijuana is a versatile and multidimensional plant, capable of being grown, processed, and consumed in many different ways. These traits are what make marijuana such a fascinating plant, with untold potential for new varieties or applications. But marijuana's versatility also presents a business opportunity for the big industries, each of which may be capable of a wholesale takeover of the marijuana industry. In part, Big Marijuana may seem like an inevitable destination because there are so many roads that can take us there.

But that doesn't mean other destinations don't exist. The legal marijuana industry is brand-new, and policymakers are scrambling to write the rules. Now is the time to think about what those rules should look like. So far, most of the rules are focused on how marijuana is sold and consumed. That makes sense, of course, since public health concerns were a primary reason marijuana was prohibited in the first place. But many other steps have to be taken before marijuana can be sold or consumed, and it all starts at the beginning of the supply chain, where farmers plant, care for, and harvest marijuana.

The agricultural sector of the marijuana industry has received far less regulatory attention. States know they have to consider how (and by whom) marijuana can be sold, as well as where (and by whom) it can be consumed. And, naturally, politicians are all too happy to devote themselves to the study of marijuana taxation. Marijuana agriculture, on the other hand, is more easily ignored or misunderstood. New York's medical marijuana law refers to the process of growing marijuana plants as "manufacturing."[9] The law doesn't say much about the "manufacturing" process, other than a requirement that plants be grown indoors.[10] That is a curious (if not uncommon) mandate for a plant that has enjoyed success being grown outdoors for thousands of years.

After Colorado voters legalized recreational marijuana use in 2012, the state created a task force to propose rules and regulations for marijuana. The recommendations the task force came up with identified some agricultural issues (such as the need to tax farmers),[11] but the more fundamental questions facing marijuana farmers (including how marijuana can be grown) went unanswered. California is no stranger to this phenomenon. Despite legalizing medical marijuana in 1996—further fueling the state's already robust marijuana farming industry—lawmakers completely neglected the subject of marijuana agriculture for twenty years. The state acted as if marijuana appeared out of thin air.

In this policy vacuum, the Big Marijuana prophecy is thriving. Despite acknowledging that no big alcohol or tobacco firms had shown an interest in the marijuana industry, the *Economist*'s cover story on marijuana on February 13, 2016, claimed that "big companies are likely to emerge," with "big farms supplying a national market." Chris Walsh, the editor of the *Marijuana Business Daily*, feels tension in the air: "I think there's a ton of paranoia that they're buying up warehouses and signing secret deals."[12]

There's no question that entrepreneurs are lining up to capitalize on the bonanza of marijuana legalization. By some measures, marijuana was already the country's most lucrative cash crop even *before* serious legalization efforts began. Surely there is money to be made in cultivating marijuana, and there are people willing to cultivate it. But is Big Marijuana inevitable? Is it beyond doubt that a few big farms will supply a national market with cheap, generic marijuana? If it isn't, what will marijuana agriculture look like? Or perhaps the better question is, what *should* marijuana agriculture look like?

These are the questions I will attempt to answer in this book.

With states across the country legalizing marijuana, the prohibition era is drawing to a close. The 2016 election season may have been divisive and hotly contested, but marijuana legalization initiatives scored resounding victories across the country. There are now twenty-nine states that have legalized marijuana in some form. These states are now facing an unprecedented challenge.

A billion-dollar industry is transitioning out of the black market and into our everyday lives. And yet, because the legalization movement is pushing forward on the strength of ballot initiatives and voters' demands, lawmakers are largely unprepared for the messy task of figuring out what comes next. That's not to say the legalization debate is not worth having anymore. It is, and each state will have to confront legalization eventually. But with most states warming to the idea of marijuana legalization, now is the time to find answers to the most pressing questions facing the industry.

Jonathan Caulkins, a professor at Carnegie Melon University, is not afraid to point out the consequences of failure: "We are going, in the United States, to legalize marijuana nationally … and there's a good chance that people in 25 to 40 years will look back and shake their heads and ask, 'What were you thinking? Why did you think it was a good idea to create an industry of titans?'"[13]

Now is the time to think about what marijuana agriculture should look like. Now is the time to ensure that the marijuana farm of the future is the type of farm Americans want it to be.

Before we think about what that farm should look like, though, we have to deconstruct the Big Marijuana prophecy. If Big Marijuana is inevitable (from an agricultural point of view, anyway), designing an alternative future will be an exercise in vain. So that is what the first part of this book will do: deconstruct the Big Marijuana prophecy, tracing the evolution of marijuana farming in America from the early days of prohibition to the modern, sophisticated agriculture practiced by today's small-scale farmers.

If you've read the title of this book, you already have a sense of what my surface conclusion is—Big Marijuana is not inevitable. That's because the

Big Marijuana prophecy relies on a number of questionable assumptions I explore in this book. To be clear, I don't mean to suggest that Big Marijuana is impossible. Nor am I suggesting that the market for marijuana can't support a diversity of agricultural products. You can enjoy a cold, light, cheap beer in one context, and a flavorful local microbrew in another context. The marijuana industry may take a similar trajectory. But it's increasingly clear that if Americans want the market to provide agricultural products that are locally and sustainably grown, the market needs to support farmers with the investments and regulations that make it all possible. And making it all possible starts with believing it is possible in the first place. That's where a deconstruction of the Big Marijuana prophecy comes in.

To begin with, the prophecy assumes that the marijuana plant is capable of large-scale cultivation. Put differently, if a few large farms are going to supply a national market, the marijuana plant must be capable of producing huge yields while maintaining a reasonable standard of quality.

It's not clear that is the case. Marijuana is a notoriously high-maintenance plant, and farmers often make adjustments to the plant's cultivation plan after daily monitoring and evaluation. As the plant grows, for example, its branches need to be tucked or supported in optimal positions, and care must be taken to give each plant just the right amount of water (too much water leads to root and stem rot; not enough water stunts plant growth). Dozens of these types of decisions must be made on a daily basis; over the course of the growing season, thousands of adjustments are made. Expertise and attention are required to produce a quality product. Fail to provide both and your chances of a successful harvest are slim.

Of course, as the marijuana industry matures, cultivation methods will too. Some mechanization of the process is likely, and innovation is to be expected. Intrepid farmers will find ways to increase yields without sacrificing too much in quality. Still, marijuana agriculture—both an art and a science at this point—looks more like the cultivation of grapevines than the growing of corn. To make matters worse for Big Marijuana hopefuls, "marijuana" is just a catch-all term for the hundreds of individual strains of the *cannabis* plant genus. Each strain has unique cultivation needs and yields a unique product. Controlling the market by flooding it with generic marijuana will be difficult when the market hasn't established a generic product to begin with.

Nonetheless, let's go ahead and assume that palatable marijuana can be grown on a large scale. The Big Marijuana prophecy also rests on the assumption that free market principles will, over time, promote a Big Marijuana model for the industry. If a few large farms are capable of flooding the market with cheap marijuana, small-scale farmers will be unable to stay competitive. Those farmers will go out of business, and the market will inevitably consolidate. The economic principles that support this process are sound. The problem is, there's no guarantee that state governments will allow the marijuana industry to operate in a completely free market environment. In fact, the early record suggests that governments see a need to protect the small-scale marijuana farmer.

In California, Lieutenant Governor Newsom's 2015 report on marijuana policy recommended "a highly regulated market ... not an unregulated free market; this industry should not be California's next Gold Rush." Furthermore, "the goal should be to prevent the growth of a large, corporate marijuana industry dominated by a small number of players." Instead, the state should look for ways to spread the economic opportunities of the new legal market: "it would be appropriate for the state to adopt laws or regulations that either encourage more small entities, or even go further, and limit the size of any individual actor involved in cultivation." If the state adopts the right mix of policies, "even small farmers should be able to operate at a scale and with a profit margin to succeed economically," the report concludes.[14]

Newsom observed that an industry composed of many small-scale farmers will probably lead to higher costs for regulators and consumers. California, at least, appears willing to pay up. Several months after the report was published, Governor Jerry Brown signed into law the Medical Marijuana Regulation and Safety Act (MMRSA), California's first meaningful attempt to regulate the marijuana industry in the twenty years since medical marijuana was legalized in the state. The MMRSA set strict limits on how large a marijuana farm could be. The maximum? Just 1 acre of marijuana plant canopy. Compare that to non-marijuana cropland in the United States, 50 percent of which is located on farms with at least 1,100 acres.[15] Even some of Jack's small-scale farming friends thought the MMRSA's acreage limits were a tad aggressive. Still, California is the country's largest producer of marijuana, and appears to have some of the best land in the country for growing it. Placing acreage limits on marijuana cultivation dealt a potentially huge blow to the Big Marijuana prophecy.

The author of the MMRSA's farming rules was Assemblyman Jim Wood, who represents the Emerald Triangle and, like other politicians who represent small-scale farming communities, is working to enact laws to protect them. In California, at least, we can expect this trend to continue. There are an estimated 50,000 marijuana farms in the state of California alone, and 30,000 of those are located in the Emerald Triangle, where the economy is dependent on marijuana agriculture. Compare that to the state's more visible wineries, of which there are only 4,000.

Farming communities are a powerful constituency, and now that the fear of prosecution is subsiding, marijuana farmers are becoming more vocal—and more organized—in their attempts to shape agricultural policy. In Humboldt County, farmers played an instrumental role in crafting the first Marijuana Ordinance. The ordinance creates farming rules at a local level, with limits on farm size, water, and energy use. It protects the small-scale farmer, certainly, but it also ensures that small-scale farming remains sustainable. In Mendocino County, farmers are organizing themselves into appellations (akin to the wine industry) designed to legally protect and promote marijuana grown in each microregion of the county.

We should expect the small-scale marijuana farming community to fight back against a Big Marijuana takeover, and we should expect their elected representatives to fight with them. There is little reason to believe that the future of the marijuana industry will be forfeited by those with the most to lose. Of course, the reverse is true as well—small-scale farmers can expect to face resistance and disruption from big businesses maneuvering for a piece of the pie. California may have struck a preemptive blow against Big Marijuana, but other states are not as prepared for the legalization era. States without many marijuana farmers, for example, don't have a constituency to protect in the first place. On the contrary, making it easy for Big Marijuana to set up shop might be an easy way for a state to compete with California's agricultural dominance.

In 2016, Oregon, Washington, and Colorado removed residency requirements for marijuana businesses, opening the door for outside investors to walk in and scale up the industry. Lifting the residency requirements was at least partly motivated by competition from California's marijuana farmers. The sponsor of the Colorado bill believed "there's only so many people willing to invest in this risky and new industry, so allowing people from out of state to become investors in this business ... seems like a good idea."[16]

After Oregon and Washington lifted their residency requirements, the *Los Angeles Times* was quick to issue the headline "How New Rules in Two

States Could Give Birth to Big Marijuana."[17] That's probably a sensational interpretation. All three states (Colorado included) continue to control the licensing process that determines how many farmers can cultivate marijuana and how much they can cultivate. Yet, while the Big Marijuana prophecy still exists, the marijuana industry is clearly still in flux. The marijuana farm of the future may or may not look like Jack's family-farming idyll, but the early record of legal marijuana farming in America gives us reason to doubt that a big business, large-scale farming takeover is inevitable.

So the good news is that there's still time to shape the marijuana industry and to create a future for marijuana agriculture that resembles a best-case scenario. With that in mind, why not make peace with Big Marijuana? After years of prohibition, some consumers might find it appealing to have marijuana abundantly available, and at the lowest price possible. Allen St. Pierre, the former director of the National Organization for the Reform of Marijuana Laws (NORML, a legalization advocacy group), sees the potential for big corporations to provide cheap marijuana to the masses, and has been meeting with corporate executives to chart a path forward. "What do we want? We can get it down to four words, almost a Wal-Mart bumper sticker: 'Best product, lowest cost,'" he said.[18]

Unfortunately, it's unlikely that Big Marijuana can provide both. Certainly, if the goal is to create marijuana products at the lowest possible cost, a Big Marijuana model is the best bet. Not everyone subscribes (or can afford to subscribe) to the idea that our agricultural products should be organic or locally grown. Marijuana consumers are a diverse bunch, and many consume marijuana for legitimate medical purposes. There is merit in providing a medical product to society at a cost that is affordable for all.

But the Big Marijuana model comes with tradeoffs. In exchange for cheap agricultural products, quality and sustainability likely have to be sacrificed. Take, for example, the Big Marijuana barons of the prohibition era: Mexican drug cartels. As recently as 2008, two-thirds of marijuana consumed in the United States came from Mexico.[19] For decades the cartels prospered by farming vast quantities of marijuana, smuggling it across the border, and selling it to American consumers. The marijuana was low in quality (known colloquially as "brick weed" or "ditch weed" due to the prevalence of chemicals, stems, seeds, and other impurities), but that didn't matter much to consumers who didn't have any other options.

Now that farmers across the United States are cultivating high-quality marijuana, the tables have turned. Border seizures of marijuana have been in decline since 2009, corroborating evidence in Mexico that cartels are struggling to adapt to consumers' preference for quality, not quantity.[20] In 2015 the U.S. Drug Enforcement Administration took notice of the shift: "Marijuana is smuggled into the United States from Mexico in large volumes ... is typically classified as 'commercial-grade' or 'low-grade' ... [and] is thought to be inferior to the marijuana produced domestically in the United States."[21]

In response, the DEA notes that "Mexican cartels are attempting to produce higher-quality marijuana to keep up with US demand."[22] So far they don't seem to have found a successful recipe: border seizures suggest the cartels have scaled down their marijuana operations, and are now focused on supplying cheap meth and heroin instead.[23] In fact, the DEA has recently observed cartels *importing* marijuana from the United States.[24] Apparently, American consumers aren't the only ones with a preference for quality weed.

Big Marijuana in the post-prohibition era could probably do better than the cartels at producing respectable marijuana in bulk (they certainly couldn't do much worse). But the downfall of the cartels' marijuana business does tell us that although growing marijuana in large quantities is possible, a quality product should not be expected. It also tells us that today's consumers prefer higher-quality marijuana, even if it comes at a higher price. Finally, it tells us that profitably growing quality marijuana in large quantities is not easy; otherwise the cartels would have adjusted to the market by now.

Here in America, our experience with food and agriculture paints a similar picture. Since World War II, the rise of massive single-crop farms and animal production facilities has slashed the cost of food and meat. But Americans have a growing awareness of the impact on public health and the environment, and popular culture increasingly expresses our concern about the industrialization of our food systems. Rachel Carson first drew national attention to the issue and spurred a new social movement when her 1962 book *Silent Spring* exposed the danger of pesticide use on our crops. More recently, diet regimens (paleo, vegan, raw, low carb, high carb), food movements (fair trade, eat local, eat organic), and alternative business models (co-ops, community-supported agriculture, meal kit delivery) pop up with regularity, catering to Americans' dissatisfaction with the status quo.

Public figures such as first lady Michelle Obama, comic John Oliver, or chef Anthony Bourdain have implored us to reevaluate our relationship with the foods we eat. Many of us have, and food industry titans from General Mills to McDonald's are slowly making changes in an attempt to hold on to their market share. In 2015 the *New York Times* described Americans' new approach to food a "seismic shift in how people eat." Researchers at New York University and Columbia argued that if big food companies don't make a fundamental shift in their approach, including a "complete overhaul of their supply chains," they won't survive.[25]

Given these trends, it's fair to wonder if the large-scale, monoculture model will work for the marijuana industry. If people want their food to be local, sustainable, and wholesome, it's likely they'll want their marijuana to be local, sustainable, and wholesome as well. Small-scale marijuana farmers can provide that; Big Marijuana probably can't. Even if decent marijuana could be cultivated in large quantities, it would probably require huge amounts of energy, pesticides, or both. Sure, there's still a market for cheap foods, and that market may carry over to the marijuana industry. But the trend is away from consolidated agriculture, and small-scale marijuana farmers are trending in the same direction.

I mentioned earlier that some politicians have argued against marijuana legalization because they fear a Big Marijuana takeover. That appears to be more than a rhetorical appeal. Lawmakers are genuinely worried that Big Marijuana will become so powerful that companies and their lobbyists will take control of the political process and aggressively promote marijuana use, making it harder for the state to keep the industry in check. Massachusetts's political leaders, for example, are afraid of powerful backers that will put "profits over people" by manipulating marijuana science and public opinion. "Preventing Another Big Tobacco" has even become the official slogan of a leading marijuana prohibition advocacy group.[26]

The California approach to marijuana agriculture—designed to limit large-scale farming operations—is partly motivated by the same concern. According to the Newsom report, "the experience of tobacco and alcohol control shows that large corporations with resources for political influence (legislative lobbying, campaign contributions, regulatory interference) and marketing muscle will promote widespread and heavy use to increase sales and profits. Legislative behavior in this context is often incongruent with public health goals." Sure enough, California's 2016 ballot initiative that legalized recreational marijuana use—backed by Silicon Valley executives—created a new farming license. Holders of this new license will be allowed to cultivate an unlimited quantity of marijuana. The provision has not received much attention, but it could have profound consequences on the marijuana industry's trajectory.

Concentrating marijuana agriculture in the hands of a few also has opportunity costs. If done right, marijuana legalization has the potential to revitalize the American family farm and rural economies nationwide. This is, after all, a billion-dollar industry, and possibly the most lucrative cash crop in the country. Many people might be uncomfortable with the mainstreaming of marijuana, but spreading the opportunities and benefits around might make it easier for us to make peace with the industry, and look forward to where it's going.

So, if Big Marijuana is neither inevitable nor the future we want, what future *do* we want? What would a marijuana industry supported by small-scale farming look like? These are the questions I explore in this book. To be more specific, there are four big questions that have not been answered:

- How should marijuana farming be organized and protected?
- Should marijuana be cultivated indoors, outdoors, or both?
- Can marijuana be cultivated with minimal impact to the environment and human health?
- Can marijuana farmers and industrial hemp farmers thrive together?

Let's think about each of these for a moment.

The answer to the first question will require some assistance from lawmakers, who have the power to make protections legally binding. But farmers and consumers can start the process by laying the foundation for the industry's organizational structure. I'll argue that the best way to organize marijuana farmers is by creating marijuana appellations. The appellation model is best known in the context of wine—when a wine label says the wine is from Napa County, you can be confident it actually came from Napa County. Similarly, "champagne" can only be affixed to the labels of sparkling wines that come from Champagne, France. If you're a wine connoisseur, you also know that some appellations (those in France, for example) have rules that dictate how, when, and which grapes can be grown in the region.

Appellations can add value to the marijuana industry in several ways. From the perspective of the local marijuana farmer, appellations provide a legally protected designation of origin. That adds value to Jack's marijuana, because it becomes a more unique product (in his case, "Humboldt County marijuana"). Jack doesn't have to worry about Big Marijuana flooding the market with a cheaper version of his product, because the products would no longer be the same. In this sense, appellations might also lend the marijuana industry a sense of sophistication that is lacking at the moment (and surely that can't hurt).

Appellations also provide a mechanism for farmers to get together and work out their local issues. In France, appellation control boards discuss and create rules designed to maintain quality standards or their product's distinguishing characteristics. The rules are often gleaned from experience and shared for mutual benefit. Since marijuana farming in America has been illegal for so long, there's been little communication between (and among) farmers and their communities. But the first marijuana appellation in the country is now taking shape in Mendocino County, California, where farmers have been refining a map of the county's microregions and setting up control boards to govern them. Now that prohibition is coming to an end, many farmers are becoming more involved and showing leadership on important issues. Appellations can keep that momentum going.

For consumers, appellations provide more transparency and protection. In the prohibition era, most marijuana transactions took place on the street (so to speak), and consumers typically had no idea where their marijuana came from. Chances were good that it came from Mexico and its sale supported cartels and drug violence, a less-than-comforting thought consumers probably didn't want to know. But now that American farmers are supplying consumers with quality marijuana, a certified designation of origin provides some measure of transparency by relaying important information (which could include the marijuana's psychoactive characteristics) to the consumer. Most people would prefer to support their local farmer instead of a nefarious cartel, and appellations can make that preference a reality.

Designations of origin also mean more options for the consumer. The number of products available multiplies as appellations add a layer of differentiation. For some consumers, that might not matter much (returning to the wine analogy, you don't need to know where a bottle of wine comes from in order to enjoy it). For others, appellations make it easier to explore and find marijuana that suits their needs. Making the place of origin significant can also promote agrotourism, a win-win for consumers and farmers. And if appellations do more than certify the place of origin—by, for example, establishing cultivation or sustainability standards—the quality of marijuana is likely to increase. Appellations are not a panacea, and present several challenges for marijuana farmers that I'll address later, but if small-scale, sustainable marijuana farming is where the industry wants to be, appellations might provide the organizational structure to get it there.

The next question—*should marijuana be cultivated indoors, outdoors, or both?*—is admittedly a contentious one. At the moment, it is a matter of considerable existential debate within the marijuana farming community, and that debate is far from settled. It is clear that marijuana can be cultivated both indoors and out. Indoor cultivation gained prominence during the prohibition era, when a basement or warehouse grow could more easily be hidden from the prying eyes of law enforcement. At the same time, outdoor cultivation thrived in places like northern California, where the remote and rugged landscape provided its own blanket of security. But which method represents the long-term solution?

The answer might depend on whether or not appellations gain acceptance. Designations of origin make sense for the wine industry in part because grapevines take on the unique characteristics of their environment (known collectively as the *terroir*). So when a connoisseur drinks a glass of wine from the northern Rhône region of France, she might detect the influence of the region's rocky soils or continental climate. There is evidence that marijuana takes on the terroir of its environment as well, another reason an appellation model is intriguing. But clearly, the terroir is less detectable if the marijuana is grown indoors, where the environmental conditions (such as the soil, light exposure, temperature, humidity, and water supplies) are tightly controlled and artificially produced. Indoor cultivation can still play a role in a market with marijuana appellations (some farmers have insisted to me that the terroir can be reproduced in an indoor environment), but outdoor farming would be a more natural fit.

That's not to say indoor cultivation doesn't have its benefits—or passionate advocates. Politicians and law enforcement authorities appreciate that it keeps marijuana farming out of sight. And farmers are more in control of the crop cycle, with no need to worry about what Mother Nature might have in store for them. They can blast grow lights at their plants day or night, through all four seasons. This method of cultivation has made it possible to push the limits of marijuana farming, driving potency levels ever higher, and allowing experimentation with hybrid strains. As nice as it is to grow crops in California, the reality is that many states don't have the growing conditions needed to satisfy the notoriously finicky marijuana plant. If we want our marijuana farming to be local, some of it will have to take place indoors.

On the other hand, there's a very good reason most crops are grown under the sun: it provides light energy for free. Other growing conditions, like the soil and climate, are also readily available. It's not as easy to control those conditions, but it's not as expensive—or energy-intensive—as reproducing them. Those costs can be staggering, and indoor cultivation might not remain profitable in the post-prohibition era when so many other farmers are growing outdoors. Eventually, when the prohibition-era barriers to interstate commerce come down, I expect the marijuana farm of the future will be an outdoor one. But until then, indoor and outdoor farmers will need to coexist.

Of course, economics and aesthetics aren't all that's at stake in this debate. Now that marijuana farming is taking place in plain sight, the environmental impacts of cultivation are coming to light. Indoor farms came under scrutiny first. A 2012 study found that the energy consumed by indoor marijuana grows (used to power lighting, ventilation, and climate control systems) alone constitutes 1 percent of total electricity use in the United States. In California, indoor cultivation accounted for 3 percent of total electricity use.[27] In Colorado, indoor marijuana farms make up over half of new demand for power.[28] While these figures remain rough estimates, it is clear that indoor farming is a highly energy-intensive production method.

Some governments have started cracking down, requiring indoor farms to produce their own renewable energy or pay higher taxes on their utility bills. Others are hoping they can incentivize farmers to be more energy efficient. "Diesel Dope" has emerged as the phrase of choice for anyone seeking to disparage indoor marijuana. If farmers want to shake that image, they will have to develop a cultivation method that is more in line with twenty-first-century sustainability standards.

But all farmers have to reckon with the environmental impacts of their trade, outdoor marijuana farmers included. Their challenge, as is often the case in the agriculture sector, is water. In March 2015, the first credible study of the impacts of marijuana cultivation on water resources found that the demand for water to irrigate marijuana plants often outstripped water supplies.[29] The study was authored by California Department of Fish and Wildlife officials, and their data came from the Eel River watershed in northern California. Shortly after the study was published, a convoy of local law enforcement vehicles drove into the remote and rugged slopes of the Eel River watershed.[30] The enforcement officers raided farmers' lands, and by the end of the week, Operation Emerald Tri-County had confiscated 86,578 marijuana plants.[31]

This time the enforcement officers were not joined by federal officials like the DEA; they were joined by the California Department of Fish and Wildlife, who suspected that many farmers didn't have permits to take water from the Eel River. Later the three counties claimed the raid itself was motivated by violations of state water regulations, not by marijuana cultivation. The operation sent a clear message to the farming community: even if marijuana use is becoming legal, marijuana farming won't get a free pass into the legal marketplace.

Farmers across the Emerald Triangle were spooked by the raid. Some of the farmers whose plants were confiscated were members of advocacy groups trying to make marijuana farming more sustainable. Others were voluntary participants in a water quality program organized by a different state agency, and now they wondered if that agency could still be trusted. Jack was in the midst of his first season on the farm, and he couldn't afford to get wiped out. His land had water rights, but getting verification from the state was risky. "If I invite them onto the property to make inspections, how do I know they won't turn around and report me?"

Many states don't have a plan for dealing with the environmental issues related to growing marijuana, and consumers are starting to feel the pain. Like any other agricultural product, organic marijuana enjoys a robust demand. Unfortunately, the term "organic" is federally regulated, and can't be used to certify marijuana products. States haven't done much to create an alternative certification or to encourage safe pesticide use. As a result, some marijuana products are being labeled as "organic," "all-natural," or "earth-friendly" when the reality is that they are anything but.

Whitney Cranshaw, an entomologist, is incredulous. In a 2015 interview, he lamented, "The Feds have completely abrogated their responsibility and let the situation devolve into chaos. [The pesticide] Avid is being used; the other big one is Floramite; and the one I really don't get is imidacloprid, which I can't even understand why you would use on this crop—it actually makes the mites worse. But the growers don't know what they're doing."[32] It might be a while before the feds can step in. Until then, states will have to fix these problems on their own.

Toward the end of this book, I'll make a concession. Although Big Marijuana might not be the future we want for the marijuana industry, Big Hemp might have some potential for the industrial hemp industry. The plant species *Cannabis sativa* can be bred to cultivate psychoactive or medicinal marijuana strains, but it can also be bred to cultivate industrial hemp. (The nomenclature of the marijuana/cannabis industry is as yet unsettled. In this book, I refer to the *cannabis* plant's psychoactive strains as "marijuana"; to the nonpsychoactive, nonmedicinal fibrous strains as "hemp"; and to all strains collectively or generally as "cannabis.") Hemp can be used to produce foods and beverages, textiles, paper, cosmetic products, insulation materials, and even energy.[33] It is one of the most versatile crops in the world, is relatively easy to grow in large quantities, and has modest environmental impacts. Even our founding fathers were quite fond of hemp. George Washington, Thomas Jefferson, and John Adams were hemp farmers, and the Declaration of Independence of the United States was drafted on hemp paper.

If Big Agriculture wants to embrace industrial hemp, the marijuana industry should be able to live with that. Hemp is already a globally traded commodity, so why not let American farmers have a turn? One problem, unfortunately, is cross-fertilization. Hemp can only be grown and sold as such if it has low levels of the psychoactive chemicals found in marijuana. In marijuana's case, female plants grow the seedless buds that get harvested and sold for consumption only if they aren't fertilized by male plants. If a hemp crop and a marijuana crop are grown in proximity to each other, they could cross-fertilize and lead to mutual destruction (from the farmer's point of view, anyway). As both crops enter the legal marketplace, farming regions across the country will have to decide which cannabis crop—marijuana or industrial hemp—they want to identify with and embrace. Both options are solid, but organization and cooperation—themes throughout this book—will be crucial. At the moment, many lawmakers and the marijuana industry haven't even begun to ask many of these important questions.

I've returned to Jack's farm several times in the past couple of years, including once for the 2015 grape harvest. It was Jack's first as the viticulturist of his own vineyard, and I could sense he was a bit anxious. As with the marijuana harvest, knowing when to pick your grapes is a mix of art and science. You need to measure the sugar content, pH, and acidity of your grapes, but only your senses can tell you if the appearance, feel, smell, and taste of the grapes is just right. Everyone had an opinion on the matter, even if no one had any relevant experience. After all, most of the workers were there to harvest and trim marijuana, not grapes.

But on a crisp and sunny Friday morning in early September, Jack felt it was time. For two days, everyone on the farm held a bucket and a pair of scissors. As they were picking, Jack's crew told stories, joked around, registered complaints, or just worked in silence. Bucket after bucket was emptied into a large bin, and at the end of the harvest, the grapes were crushed and destemmed. These days, crushing grapes with your feet isn't really necessary, but they did it anyway. Champagne bottles were opened (sparkling wine, technically), and Jack toasted to the conclusion of his first harvest as a farmer, beaming with pride.

Jack and his team were feeling their way through a new agricultural experience. The grape harvest wasn't perfectly executed, of course, but they were capable farmers, with the right tools and mentality for the job. Like Jack, this country is feeling its way through a new agricultural experience as well. We don't have easy answers for the tough questions facing the marijuana industry. But we do have the right tools and mentality for the job. The opportunity is there for us to make sure the marijuana farm of the future is the marijuana farm we want it to be. Let's take advantage of it.

2 A Brief History of Marijuana Farming

Seems to me if grate Men dont leeve off writing Pollyticks, breaking Heads, boxing Ears, ringing Noses and kicking Breeches, we shall by and by want a world of Hemp more for our own consumshon.
—John Adams, second president of the United States

Agriculture is now, as it's always been, the basis of civilization. The 6 million farms of the United States ... form the basis of all other achievements of the American people, and are more fruitful than all their other resources.
—Theodore Roosevelt, twenty-sixth president of the United States

Humans have been around for some 200,000 years,[1] and for most of that period our ancestors were nomadic hunter-gatherers. Populations were small, mobile, and opportunistic.[2] They were heavily influenced by availability of food and water, responding quickly to changes in their surrounding environment. Frequently on the move, humans weren't able to accumulate vast troves of resources or possessions. But, as a result of this adaptable, nomadic lifestyle, hunter-gatherers learned to thrive in diverse habitats. Eventually (around 35,000 years ago) humans inhabited much of the Eastern Hemisphere, from France to Australia, and Africa to Siberia.[3]

Humans didn't start cultivating crops until around ten thousand years ago, which makes agriculture a relatively modern technology. Near the end of the last ice age, the retreat of snow and ice unlocked fertile lands surrounding large river systems. With constant water sources and productive soils, these lands could support human life year-round. It wasn't long before humans started manipulating local plants to make them grow productively near their settlements. This agricultural discovery—known as the Neolithic Revolution—transformed human society as we knew it. Previously nomadic communities became settled. Locally available plants and animals were domesticated, cultivated, and, eventually, traded throughout the world. Surplus food production allowed for population growth, labor specialization, private property ownership, and the accumulation and concentration of wealth and political power.

In order to maximize productivity, farmers concentrated on growing large quantities of a select number of plants. Tastes became more discerning and focused than those of our hunter-gatherer predecessors. Only the most useful plants would be worth cultivating, and those were often plants that were highly productive, resilient, nutritious, or versatile. Some of the earliest crops (known as "Neolithic founder crops") included cereals (wheat and barley), legumes (lentils and peas), and flax.[4] Many of these plants can be used for food or fiber, and are relatively easy to store and sell.

Cannabis has much in common with the founder crops. It, too, can be used for food or fiber (in addition to medicinal and psychoactive uses), and can grow in conditions unsuitable to other vegetation. It might not be surprising, then, that there is increasing evidence to suggest that cannabis was also one of the first plant species to be cultivated by humans. Some scholars believe cannabis may have helped bring about the Neolithic Revolution in the first place.[5]

The cannabis plant is naturally adapted to open spaces and sunny climates, preferring nitrogen-rich soils. Clearings and waste sites created by camps of hunter-gatherers could have produced ideal growing conditions. Once discovered, the plant's strong fibers and nutritious seeds would have been valued and harvested, providing opportunities for cannabis to take root in or near the camp, and eventually bridging the gap between gathering and farming. From there, it is not difficult to imagine that the medicinal and psychoactive properties of cannabis would be unlocked by fire and incorporated into spiritual traditions.

Cannabis would have been an excellent plant for early agriculturalists to experiment with and use to hone their horticultural manipulation skills. Depending on their community's needs and the demands of the market, early farmers may have preferred cannabis strains that were preternaturally fibrous, seedy, psychoactive, or medicinal, launching the practice of plant breeding that continues to this day.

Chinese botanist Hui-Lin Li wrote in 1974 that cannabis is "one of man's oldest cultivated crops."[6] Because humans have cultivated cannabis for such a long time, it is not clear where the plant originated. Cultivation and trade would have hastened its geographic spread and fostered the growth of feral plants in wild, nonnative habitats, obscuring its true origin. Yet cannabis most likely originated somewhere in Asia. Different scholars have suggested that the plant may be native to Central Asia, South Asia, or East Asia.[7] Russian botanist Nikolai Vavilov suggested in the 1940s that each of these regions may have been an independent center of cannabis origin, yielding the three major categories of cannabis plants: fibrous hemp plants in East Asia, psychoactive or medicinal plants in South Asia, and nutritious food plants in Central Asia.[8] Vavilov's theory has been questioned as being too simplistic, but a definitive answer remains elusive.

Still, archaeological evidence supports the idea that humans have cultivated cannabis since Neolithic times. Ancient China's history with cannabis farming is so ingrained that for some time the region was known as "The Land of Mulberry and Hemp." The earliest evidence of cannabis cultivation is indirect: pottery with markings likely created by hemp fiber that was found along the southern China coast has been dated to 10,000 BCE.[9] Similar markings created by the Tapenkeng people circa 5000 BCE were found on the island of Taiwan.[10] Near China's Yellow River, archaeologists have been finding 4,000- to 6,000-year-old hempen impressions since the 1920s, and hemp seeds since the 1980s.[11] By 1000 BCE, cannabis had become one of the most economically important and ubiquitous crops in East Asia.[12]

The prominent role cannabis farming played in ancient China was documented in China's earliest agricultural texts and promoted by some of its most prominent thinkers and agronomists. The renowned Emperor Shennong (which translates into "God Farmer" or "Agriculture God"), said to have lived 4,500 years ago, is considered the father of Chinese medicine and agriculture. He instructed farmers to grow cannabis and recommended a "hemp elixir" to treat the sick.[13] Hemp is identified as a primary agricultural crop in the oldest Chinese agricultural treatise (circa 1000 BCE), the *Xia Xiao Zheng*. *The Book of Songs and the Annals* (circa 500 BCE) named hemp one of the six commonly planted crops in China. Confucius, one of China's most influential thinkers, often wrote about hemp, providing his own insights on farming methods or quoting references to hemp farming in other literature.

While hemp cultivation in ancient China is well documented, cannabis farming has a long history in the rest of Eurasia as well. Cultivation took place as far back as Neolithic times in the Caucasus Mountains of Central Asia, the Himalaya Mountains of Afghanistan, and the Indian subcontinent.

In fact, ancient Hindu texts provide their own theory on the origin of cannabis: according to the Vedas, the seminal books of the Hindu faith (circa 1100 BCE), cannabis was brought down from the Himalayas by the god Shiva for the pleasure of humanity.[14] Buddhists were equally interested in the spiritual powers of cannabis. According to Buddhist legend, Siddhartha (who would go on to find enlightenment and become Buddha) spent six years living on an exclusive diet of one hemp seed per day.[15]

Around 2000 BCE nomadic tribes began spreading knowledge about cannabis cultivation to lands beyond Central Asia. One of these, the Aryans, introduced cannabis farming to Persia, Asia Minor, and Europe.[16] By 1500 CE, cannabis farming had spread to Africa and Southeast Asia.[17] Herodotus, the Greek historian, may have been the first European to write about cannabis in the fifth century BCE. He observed cannabis being used by cultures in Macedonia and the Balkans, largely for spiritual or psychoactive purposes. The Greeks themselves were not avid cannabis farmers at the time, but Greek scholars and doctors were making interesting discoveries that did not escape the attention of their employers, the Roman Empire.[18]

Though it took some time, the Roman Empire would come to recognize the strategic importance of domestic hemp production to supply rope and textiles for their armies and navies. The Romans relied on imports at first, trading for hemp grown in Central Asia and the hinterlands of the empire. But as the empire grew, so did the demand for hempen fibers. The risk that these imports could be cut off by foreign suppliers made Rome vulnerable, so the empire began to invest in the expansion of cannabis agriculture within its own confines.[19] Farms sprung up closer to Rome, and perhaps inevitably, cannabis farming became a military imperative of the Roman Empire.

The Romans would be far from the last great empire to encourage (or force) its own farmers to grow cannabis. In fact, the cannabis plant's ability to produce the best sails and ropes for the world's great navies hastened its cultivation throughout the world. After the fall of the Roman Empire, the Franks (known for being agriculturally advanced) took up the torch of European production. The city states of Italy also began to cultivate cannabis; they were renowned maritime traders and couldn't afford to subject their fleets to the vagaries of foreign hemp suppliers. Venice, in particular, was so successful in growing quality cannabis that it became an exporter to the rest of Europe. The Russian empire, too, recognized and seized the opportunity cannabis agriculture presented. By the seventeenth century Russia was growing so much hemp that it had become the world's largest producer, supplying 90 percent of England's demand.[20] The leverage this created over Europe's other maritime powers, suffice it to say, did not go unnoticed.

The Dutch, British, and Spanish built their colonial empires by harnessing the power of a large merchant and naval fleet. Copious amounts of cannabis were necessary to produce the sails and ropes their ships needed to withstand the rigors of global conquest. By one estimate, the English fleet that warded off the Spanish Armada may have required 10,000 acres of land for hemp production.[21] The Spanish Armada itself may have required even more. To their credit, Europe's naval powers tried to meet these demands at home. Fifty years before the Spanish Armada came to England's shores, King Henry VIII made hemp farming mandatory for every farmer in England. His daughter, Queen Elizabeth I, doubled down on her father's bold policy by increasing the fine for noncompliance.

Yet even these policies didn't produce enough hemp, as Western Europe was too crowded to support widespread cannabis farming. With the Russians continuing to dominate the global hemp trade, the Europeans looked westward. In the New World, arable land was limitless, and colonial labor cheap. The Spanish introduced and encouraged cannabis farming in Peru, Colombia, Chile, Mexico, and California, where large hemp farms emerged on the outskirts of Los Angeles and San Francisco.[22] The French did the same in Quebec, "encouraging" farmers to grow hemp by seizing and withholding textiles from those who refused.

The British were even more domineering with their American colonies. In fact, before Jamestown was founded in 1607, one contractual requirement of settlement included the cultivation of hemp by the colonists. In a sense, then, American cannabis farming predates colonial America itself. And matters quickly escalated. By 1619 every colonist in Virginia (farmer or not) was required to grow at least 100 plants. Connecticut and Massachusetts imposed similar requirements not long after. Hemp became legal tender to pay taxes and debts.

These policies succeeded in turning colonial America into a cannabis-growing force, but the demand for hemp in the colonies was so great that very little supply made its way back to Britain. Naturally, this result inflamed the British, who passed laws prohibiting hemp weaving and wool imports with the hope these measures would make the colonies reliant on British textile manufacturers.[23] Predictably, however, they only served to make the colonists more self-sufficient. Tensions over the rise of the American hemp textile industry became a cause of the American Revolutionary War, as well as a factor in its ultimate resolution.

The cannabis plant played a major role in the founding and expansion of the United States. As mentioned in chapter 1, drafts of the Declaration of Independence were written on hemp paper. In the years following the Revolutionary War, state and federal currencies competed with each other for monetary credibility. The price of hemp being more stable, hemp became a currency safety net, functioning much as a gold standard might. For a time, hemp was even a pioneer crop, providing food, fiber, and fuel for settlers heading west.

Many of our founding fathers were cannabis farmers. George Washington was an avid hemp farmer before and during his presidency. His diary entries during the pre-presidential years are replete with his own observations of hemp growth and farming methods. As president, Washington sent letters to his estate manager with instructions for cultivating hemp. He may even have been one of the first Americans to be seduced by the many strains of cannabis:

> What was done with the Seed saved from the India Hemp last Summer? It ought, *all* of it, to have been sown again; that not only a stock of seed sufficient for my own purposes might have been raised, but to have disseminated the seed to others; as it is more valuable than the common Hemp.[24]

John Adams, the second president of the United States, was more hemp advocate than farmer. As a young writer working for the *Boston Gazette* and *Boston Evening Post*, Adams encouraged readers to grow hemp, providing instructions on how to care for and harvest cannabis plants. In one passage, written under the pseudonym of Humphrey Ploughjogger, he appeared to recognize the medicinal potential of cannabis: "Seems to me if grate Men dont leeve off writing Pollyticks, breaking Heads, boxing Ears, ringing Noses and kicking Breeches, we shall by and by want a world of Hemp more for our own consumshon."[25] Adams's devotion to hemp farming was maintained into his political years. In January 1776, Adams wrote a two-page to-do list on his way to the Continental Congress, with items such as "forces to be raised" and "taxes to be laid and levied." Scroll down the list and you'll find that "hemp to be encouraged" made it to page one. You won't find "Declaration of Independency" until the bottom of page two.

John Adams's rival and presidential successor, Thomas Jefferson, was equally (if not more) invested in cannabis agriculture. Jefferson's agricultural estate included 5,000 acres of farmland, much of which was devoted to tobacco in his early years. Eventually, however, Jefferson would pivot toward hemp. Although he notes that hemp cultivation methods at the time were "so slow, so laborious, and so much complained of by our laborers" that he had to give it up for a while (not to be taken lightly, since those "laborers" he refers to were slaves), Jefferson too recognized that hemp farming was in the national interest:

> The fact well established in the system of agriculture is that the best hemp and the best tobacco grow on the same kind of soil. The former article is of first necessity to the commerce and marine, in other words to the wealth and protection of the country. The latter, never useful and sometimes pernicious, derives its estimation from caprice, and its value from the taxes to which it was formerly exposed.[26]

Hemp thereafter became one of the most important agricultural crops in the United States. Particularly in the South, where slave labor could be used to overcome the rigors of the harvest, hemp farming flourished. Hemp was of such value, and its cultivation at the time so demanding, that hemp-farming slaves were some of the most expensive on the market. Some even managed to parlay their toils and expertise into paid positions, in some cases making enough to buy their freedom.[27]

Despite technological advancements that made the harvest much less physically demanding, hemp cultivation declined in the late nineteenth century. American farmers were turning to other crops while foreign countries were fulfilling the domestic hemp demand. Nonetheless, hemp production in the United States remained modest but steady heading into the twentieth century.

While cannabis farming in the United States owes its birth to the nation's colonial ancestors, American farmers did their part to influence the cannabis trade as well. When American farmers began to flood world markets with good, smokable tobacco, the combination with tobacco made psychoactive marijuana much easier to smoke. Ironically, although American cannabis farming from colonial times through the nineteenth century was focused on producing fibrous hemp strains, tobacco exports spurred a global increase in the growth and consumption of psychoactive strains.

As many contemporary marijuana smokers know, fresh marijuana can be sticky and damp, as well as potent. Prior to the sixteenth century, psychoactive cannabis was primarily ingested with food or alcohol or burned on a fire to create vapors. The addition of tobacco makes it easier to light and smoke marijuana, and the nicotine high is (for some) an added benefit. The widespread availability of American-grown tobacco changed the way the world consumed cannabis. From the sixteenth century onward, hashish (psychoactive cannabis resin) and tobacco were smoked together, a practice that continues to this day in many regions of the world.

With the growth in popularity of tobacco and marijuana came a need for cannabis agriculture to focus on cultivating psychoactive strains. South Asia, where cannabis is native, ramped up its marijuana farming in the eighteenth and nineteenth centuries. Agriculture centers included Indian states such as Madhya Pradesh in central India, Kerala in the south, and West Bengal to the east.[28] The Hindu Kush mountains along the border of Pakistan and Afghanistan are considered the birthplace of a family of psychoactive marijuana strains. Farmers there, too, cultivated marijuana and spread its seeds around the world.

Greece also emerged as a marijuana-growing powerhouse in the nineteenth century. With cheap labor from the Middle East, countless sea ports to distribute the harvest, and a favorable climate, Greek farmers became prolific marijuana exporters. Thanks to Henry de Montfried, a French soldier turned hashish smuggler, we have a description of Greek marijuana farming that is eerily reminiscent of the artisanal farming scene in northern California today:

> All the farms in this district prepared hashish; it was their chief industry. Each estate had its brand, quoted on the market, and there were good and bad years, exactly as for wines.[29]

Not long after de Montfried published his account, marijuana farming in Greece was outlawed and cultivation moved to the Middle East and North Africa. This region has remained an active marijuana-growing region until recently, when military conflict and political instability have threatened agricultural markets. Morocco, Lebanon, Syria, Turkey, Iran, Iraq, and Egypt were major marijuana growing countries.[30] It is less clear today whether these countries are still actively growing marijuana, and if so, on what scale. But Morocco is still believed to be one of the world's largest hashish producers due to prolific cultivation in the wet and fertile Rif mountains of northern Morocco.[31]

Marijuana agriculture also emerged in Latin America and the Caribbean, where psychoactive strains were cultivated by native populations across Colombia, Jamaica, and Brazil. They may have been introduced to marijuana farming by migrant laborers from India and Africa, or they figured out how to cultivate psychoactive strains themselves from the hemp plants introduced by their colonizers. It wasn't long after the Spanish introduced hemp farming to Mexico that they observed native laborers smoking it, which suggests that whatever strains were being used to produce fiber were capable of being manipulated over time to produce marijuana as well.

By the beginning of the twentieth century, marijuana was being cultivated widely throughout Mexico and was starting to creep into the southern United States, as Mexican laborers brought it with them when entering the States to find work. Hemp was still being cultivated in the United States, of course, and a rising interest in the medicinal qualities of cannabis drove up the demand for domestic marijuana. But hemp farmers faced stiff competition from other textile producers, and marijuana's popularity as a recreational drug or alternative medicine was still limited. As a result, the United States was not a major agricultural producer of marijuana in the early twentieth century.

Instead, the dominant marijuana-exporting regions of the world at the turn of the twentieth century were Latin America, from Mexico to Colombia; the Middle East and North Africa, from Morocco to Afghanistan; and the South Asian trio of Pakistan, India, and Nepal. More isolated hotspots included Greece, Thailand, and Vietnam. Do-it-yourself marijuana users were also growing their own supply all over the world. Before the war on drugs put marijuana farmers firmly in its crosshairs, cannabis was being grown openly and with commercial success on every continent on earth, much as it had been for centuries.

This ancient and extensive history of cannabis farming has given rise to the idea that prohibitions put in place in the mid-twentieth century were the first of their kind—a whirlwind of racial, political, and economic forces that successfully used marijuana prohibition as a pretext for suppression. By contrasting prohibition with our ancient history of cannabis farming, some historians make our modern-day drug laws appear irregular and shortsighted. In his seminal (and controversial) book on cannabis, *The Emperor Wears No*

Clothes (referred to by many legalization advocates as "the Hemp Bible"), Jack Herer opens with the following line:

> For thousands upon thousands of years, all over the world, whole families came together to harvest the hemp fields at the height of the flowering season, never dreaming that one day the U.S. government would be spearheading an international movement to wipe the cannabis plant off the face of the earth.[32]

Yet, while unprecedented in scope, the United States' war on drugs was not the first of its kind. The reality is that marijuana has been controversial for almost as long as humans have been farming it. Many societies throughout history have banned cannabis cultivation and use. What many of these crackdowns and prohibitions have in common is social and economic inequality, or a distrust of the unknown. When members of a minority or lower class embrace marijuana use, the ruling class moves to outlaw marijuana as a form of suppression and control. Marijuana is perceived to be a threat to the order of society, and stamping it out naturally begins with a prohibition on cultivation.

As a case in point, the ancient Chinese might have been the first cannabis farmers—and, as far as we know, were the first to write about psychoactive marijuana—and yet they may also have been the first to reject it as a socially acceptable drug. The rise of Taoism around 600 BCE brought with it a cultural rejection of intoxicants. Marijuana was then viewed as antisocial, and derisively dismissed by one Taoist priest as a loony drug reserved for shamans.[33] The sentiment persisted into the modern era—to this day, marijuana struggles to disassociate itself with the stained history of opium in China.

Muslim societies have a complex relationship history with marijuana. Hashish use spread widely with the expansion of Islam in the seventh century CE, and remains popular today. Early Arabic texts referred to marijuana as the "bush of understanding" and the "morsel of thought."[34] Yet traditional theologians believed Mohammed prohibited marijuana use (the Koran [2: 219] prohibits "intoxicants," but how that word should be interpreted is still up for debate). One prominent theologian associated marijuana with the dreaded Mongol empire, and many upper-class Muslims pushed for prohibition, for fear that marijuana use would disrupt the labor force. In the end, some societies tolerated marijuana use or turned a blind eye; others (such as Damascus in 1265) embraced prohibition.

Sufi Muslims took these tensions to the next level. The mystical Sufis believed that spiritual enlightenment could be reached by an altered state of consciousness, and a mind-bending drug like marijuana would seem a logical vehicle to reach that state. Sufis believed hashish was a vehicle not only to personal enlightenment but to direct communication with Allah. These beliefs did not go over well with the rest of mainstream Islam, however. To make matters worse for the Sufis, they were often lower-class laborers. That marijuana use was therefore central to a religion perceived to be a heretical challenge to religious, economic, and political order made the plant an easy target for authorities.

In 1253, Sufis were openly growing marijuana in Cairo, Egypt. The government, claiming that Sufism was a threat to society, raided their farms and destroyed all their crops. Undeterred, the Sufis made deals with farmers in the Nile River Valley to grow marijuana on their farmlands. This successful agricultural partnership lasted until 1324, when Egyptian troops raided the countryside and destroyed all the marijuana they could find. For Sufis and marijuana farmers, the situation only got worse. Martial law was imposed in 1378, and this time the authorities destroyed more than marijuana crops: entire farms and farming villages were burned to the ground. Farmers were imprisoned or executed, and hashish users had their teeth pulled.[35] Despite this swift and vicious crackdown, the demand for hashish remained strong. The cycle of cultivation, consumption, and crackdown continued in Egypt for centuries.

Islam was not the only major world religion to feel threatened by marijuana. Pope Innocent VIII issued a papal ban on cannabis in the first year of his papacy, in 1484. At the time, marijuana, along with other mind-altering plants, was being cultivated for medicinal and spiritual applications throughout Europe by pagans who were considered to be witches and sorcerers. The Christianity of Pope Innocent VIII, however, was predicated on a future fulfillment in the afterlife, and a rejection of momentary pleasures or enlightenment. The pagans growing marijuana profoundly challenged this premise by promising spiritual enrichment in the present, with a plant grown right here on earth. Pope Innocent VIII thus wasted no time in addressing this existential threat, declaring cannabis to be an unholy sacrament of the satanic Mass. The pagans who cultivated it were persecuted into imprisonment, exile, or death.[36]

Colonial empires, with their unfailing concern for a robust military and hard-working labor force, have often viewed marijuana with suspicion. Though the Spanish were one of the first colonial empires to encourage the cultivation of hemp in the Americas, they were not as enthusiastic about marijuana. The Spanish governor of Mexico issued an order in 1550 limiting cannabis farming because "the natives were beginning to use the plant for something other than rope."[37] White South Africans, descended from Dutch or British colonialists, passed a series of laws in the nineteenth century designed to crack down on the cultivation and use of marijuana by indentured Indian farm workers, who were viewed by whites as societal contaminants and a threat to civil order.[38]

The Portuguese empire also struggled to control cannabis. The Portuguese wanted to foster a strong hemp-producing workforce just like those of their colonial rivals, but they considered marijuana a pernicious vice, especially when used by slaves. The Portuguese introduced marijuana prohibitions to many of their African colonies, including Zambia and Angola. Nonetheless, explorers to the region noticed marijuana being grown "nearly everywhere" and used by "all the tribes of the interior."[39]

When the Portuguese brought slaves to Brazil in the sixteenth century, the slaves brought marijuana along with them, as seeds were sewn into the clothing they wore onto the slave ships and then germinated upon arrival. Whatever strains they were using must have been well adapted to the Brazilian landscape; marijuana was soon growing from the coasts to the Amazon and everywhere in between.[40] For the most part, marijuana cultivation was permitted during Portuguese rule. But when Brazil gained its independence in the early nineteenth century, Rio de Janeiro's municipal cannabis prohibition started a chain reaction of prohibitions around the country aimed at curbing marijuana use among slave populations.[41]

One reason Portugal may have been lenient on marijuana farming in Brazil is the fact that the Queen of Portugal herself was using it while stationed there during the Napoleonic wars.[42] This wasn't the first time Napoleon Bonaparte was involved in the history of marijuana. Several years earlier, in 1798, Napoleon had launched the French campaign into Egypt and Syria, a large-scale offensive designed to cut off British trade and liberate Egypt from Ottoman rule. After the initial conquest, Napoleon attempted to maintain local support by embracing Islamic culture and scientific exchange. An unusually large percentage of French forces in Egypt (totaling around 40,000) were scientists and scholars, and were responsible for establishing libraries, laboratories, and research centers that went on to make significant contributions in a number of disciplines.

The discovery of hashish may not have been seen as a breakthrough at the time, but it had a great effect on European culture and literary thought. Prior to the French campaign in Egypt, hashish wasn't well known in Europe and certainly wasn't commonly used. The 40,000 French troops stationed in Egypt, however, quickly learned about it. Hashish was ubiquitous in Egypt at the time, bought and sold in cafés, markets, and smoking lounges. Lacking access to their customary French wines and liquors and encouraged by Napoleon to embrace Egyptian culture, many French troops took up hashish.

Unfortunately, hashish was still associated with Sufi mystics and looked down upon by the Sunni elite. After Napoleon went back to France, the general he had left in charge of Egypt, General Jacques-François Menou, was a noble-born French revolutionary who married into an upper-class Sunni family after taking command of Egypt. For Menou, the prospect of a hashish ban killed two birds with one stone: it would appease the Sunni elite by cracking down on Sufis, and alleviate a perceived public health problem among the French troops. The *ordre du jour* banning the cultivation, sale, and consumption of cannabis, considered by some scholars to be the first drug prohibition law in the modern era, came down in 1800. It opens with the following:

> Article One: The use of strong liquor, made by certain Muslims with a certain grass [*herbe*] called hashish, and smoking of the seed of cannabis, are prohibited throughout Egypt. Those who are accustomed to drinking this liquor and smoking this seed lose reason and fall into a violent delirium, which often leads them to commit excesses of all kinds.[43]

Whether or not Menou's order was the first modern penal law on drugs, it largely failed to work (a fact that should come as no surprise to us in the twenty-first century). Hashish continued to be produced, sold, and consumed widely throughout Egypt, and it came home with French troops when they left Egypt in 1801. It wasn't long before hashish was being widely used in France and the rest of western Europe.

Despite efforts by authorities in Europe to paint hashish as an unstable and dangerous substance,[44] many of the Romantic period's most accomplished artists and writers were brought together because of cannabis. Dubbing themselves *Le Club des Hachichins* (Hashish-Eaters' Club), luminaries such as Théophile Gautier, Charles Baudelaire, Gérard de Nerval, Victor Hugo, Honoré de Balzac, and Alexandre Dumas would meet in Paris to take hashish and exchange notes on their experiences.[45] They rejected mainstream attempts to associate hashish with what was regarded as Oriental barbarism and, through their writings, normalized marijuana use and popularized the Romantic era's bohemian creed: *l'art pour l'art* (art for art's sake).

Across the Channel, the British Empire wrestled with the conspicuous presence of cannabis in India. As a native plant to the Indian subcontinent, cannabis could be found growing in the wild by hunter-gatherers, and was likely cultivated by the earliest agrarian settlers. Psychoactive marijuana strains featured prominently in early texts of the Hindu, Buddhist, and Tantrist religions. As the Indian marijuana farming industry matured over time, the harvested product was divided into three gradients, all of which remain available today.

Bhang is the cheapest, most prevalent, and lowest-quality marijuana; it consists of crushed leaves, seeds, and/or flowers, and produces the least potent high. On the other end of the spectrum, *Charas* is the highest-quality and most expensive marijuana in India. It is sold as a highly potent hashish produced from plants grown in the most desirable cannabis-producing farmlands of the Hindu Kush and Himalaya mountain ranges between 4,000 to 7,000 feet. It remains one of the most revered marijuana products in the world today. Somewhere in between *Bhang* and *Charas* is *Ganga*. A midgrade crop in both price and potency, *Ganga* is cultivated from well-cared-for female plants, and consists of a mixture of resin and cannabis flower.[46]

One of the first Europeans to write about the Indian marijuana industry was a Portuguese doctor named Garcia da Orta. He wrote of *Bhang* in 1563:

> The Indians get no usefulness from this, unless it is in the fact that they become ravished by ecstasy, and delivered from all worries and cares, and laugh at the least little thing. After all, it is said that it was they who first found the use of it.[47]

Some two hundred years later, the British mulled over the possibility of a marijuana prohibition in India. The Indian ruling class and the British governor-general of India pushed for a total ban, fearful that marijuana would create social unrest. The British Parliament, however, had other ideas. Short on cash, the government saw the marijuana industry as an opportunity to raise some revenue. They taxed cannabis in 1790, and three years later, established a regulatory framework to issue licenses to farmers and sellers.[48]

The tax-and-regulate scheme worked to some extent. But in a vast landscape where cannabis grows in the wild, many farmers and their crops escaped the tax. The British encouraged the regulatory system to decentralize, allowing cities and states to experiment with different taxation schemes. The results were mixed. The strength of the black market was frustrating enough that the British Parliament considered prohibition measures in 1838, 1871, 1877, and 1892.[49] But ultimately the measures failed to pass, because the tax revenues that did come in couldn't be ignored.

Temperance movement advocates persisted, however, driven by the evils of opium use which they associated with cannabis. Parliament responded by commissioning the most comprehensive government study of marijuana in human history. The seven-volume 3,500-page *Report of the Indian Hemp Drugs Commission* of 1894 to 1895 called over a thousand witnesses from around the world. The findings emphatically rejected the alleged grounds for prohibition. The commission found (as its predecessors did) that marijuana cultivation is nearly impossible to eradicate, and argued that it produces no "evil results" in the first place:

> Total prohibition of the cultivation of the hemp plant for narcotics, and of the manufacture, sale, or use of the drugs derived from it, is neither necessary nor expedient in consideration of their ascertained effects, of the prevalence of the habit of using them, of the social and religious feeling on the subject, and of the possibility of its driving the consumers to have recourse to other stimulants or narcotics which may be more deleterious.[50]

The commission went on to recommend a tax-and-license scheme for the marijuana farming industry:

> The means to be adopted for the attainment of [control and restriction] are:
>
> • adequate taxation, which can be best effected by the combination of a direct duty with the auction of the privilege of vend;
>
> • prohibiting cultivation, except under license, and centralizing cultivation.[51]

This represents, to my knowledge, the first time in history a government study has recommended a centralized marijuana farming scheme. Comprehensive as it is in other respects, however, the commission's report does not elaborate on this centralization proposal; it merely suggests that the most effective way of limiting supply is "to grant licenses for cultivation in such a way as to secure supervision and registration of the produce."[52]

Despite the commission's efforts, Parliament's endorsement of its report was lukewarm. As a result, the marijuana farming trade continued unchanged, with taxation and licensing of cultivators continuing to be hit and miss. *Bhang* was informally grown nearly everywhere; *Ganga* crops were, for the most part, produced on government-licensed farms; and *Charas* was imported from the Hindu Kush and Himalayas.[53] This basic structure persisted into the global prohibition era of the twentieth century. The proposal to "centralize cultivation" was largely forgotten after the commission's report was published. But a century later, government regulators trying to find their way through the post-prohibition era of the twenty-first century would come to recognize its advantages.

The history of marijuana farming tells us that when prohibitions are imposed, they almost always come from the ruling class. Marijuana's role as a spiritual, medicinal, or recreational drug of the poor working classes stokes fears among the elite that the political, religious, or economic order that has served them so well may be disrupted. There aren't, therefore, many cases where marijuana was embraced by the ruling class and persecuted from below. But the story of the Bashilange tribe suggests that marijuana users can be targeted from any angle.

In the mid-nineteenth century, the eastern region of the Democratic Republic of the Congo in central Africa was a vast wilderness, and it was controlled by the Bashilange tribe. The Bashilange were ruthless fighters, eating the bodies of their victims and enslaving their prisoners. They enacted few laws, save a requirement that other tribes in the region pay tribute to their supremacy or face a certain death. While exploring these lands, however, the Governor of German East Africa observed a remarkable shift in the Bashilange's culture. The tribe had discovered marijuana, and rapidly embraced the plant as a pillar of their tribe's identity.

Tribesmen of the Bashilange dubbed themselves the Sons of Cannabis, and soon passed laws to promote peace and friendship. They rejected cannibalism and were no longer permitted to carry weapons in the village. They stopped killing their rivals, and started having more sex. Marijuana was smoked regularly and at most important events, including religious ceremonies, holidays, and political alliances. Formerly known for being cold-blooded killers, the Sons of Cannabis became tranquil marijuana-growing peacemakers.

Unfortunately, their rivals did not share the Sons of Cannabis's new-found love of peace and friendship. Many tribes lost respect for their former rulers and stopped making tribute payments. With weakening support in the region, the Bashilange tribe splintered. The Sons of Cannabis, no longer the fearsome fighters of yore, were overthrown by their fellow tribesmen who yearned for a return to the tribe's dominant past. The new regime reinstituted the tribe's violent practices, and largely returned the Bashilange to its former warring nature.[54]

Jack Herer may have been using hyperbole when he claimed that cannabis farmers throughout history could not have conceived of the twentieth century's crackdown on marijuana. The historical record illustrates that while many regions of the world have tolerated or embraced marijuana farming in the past, plenty of others have seen authorities attempt to exterminate farmers and their crops. Targeting the first step in the supply chain is a logical starting point for prohibitionists, and marijuana's role as an agent of religious, political, or economic change has long made it a threat to the established social order.

Our marijuana-farming ancestors of the past could have told us, based on experience, that when prohibitionists come after cannabis, they will do so in predictable ways. They will use rhetoric to associate the plant with violence, depravity, and other more dangerous drugs, as the European temperance movement did in France and Great Britain. They will use a militarized show of force to eradicate crops, persecute farmers, and dissuade the next generation from growing marijuana, as the Ottomans did in Egypt. They will portray marijuana users as religious extremists or dangerous minorities, as Pope Innocent VIII did in Europe, Sunni Muslims did in the Middle East, or white South Africans did in South Africa. The best-case scenario, they might say, is that the authorities will turn a blind eye to the unstoppable forces of supply and demand, much as the Portuguese did in Brazil or the British did in India.

In telling us this, our marijuana-farming ancestors might as well have been writing the playbook for the twentieth-century war on drugs. The cannabis prohibition era in the United States did not invent this "greatest hits" collection of tactics that prohibitionists have been using for centuries; it simply brought them all together in one place, and injected them with more financial and military resources than any prohibition movement in history has ever seen.

3   The Fall and Rise of American Marijuana Farming

I want a Goddamn strong statement on marijuana ... I mean one on marijuana that just tears the ass out of them. ... By God we are going to hit the marijuana thing, and I want to hit it right square in the puss. ... I want to hit it, against legalizing and all that sort of thing.

—Richard Nixon, thirty-seventh president of the United States[1]

The 2017 harvest was a crop to forget for Elaine. A sixty-five-year-old veteran of the war on drugs, Elaine qualifies as an old-timer in Humboldt County. She is a resilient and well-respected grower in the community, and she's experienced her share of booms and busts over the years. But 2017 felt different, as if the political forces at work in the state capital of Sacramento were blowing the winds of change in her direction, with little hope of relenting.

Marijuana grown in Humboldt County, where winter rains replenish reservoirs and summers bring the dry, sunny skies that marijuana plants thrive on, has long been considered among the best in the world. Certainly warehouse grows can produce the meticulously crafted buds that turn heads among connoisseurs on the cannabis trade show competition circuit. But the scale of production that Humboldt's tens of thousands of farms can sustain, as well as the region's reputation for quality product, are unrivaled. For decades Humboldt has been king of the American marijuana agriculture industry, with a dominance that survived sustained attacks from paramilitarized federal, state, and local law enforcement. But even the most grizzled veterans of the prohibition era are no match for the market forces of supply and demand.

In the heyday of black-market marijuana economics, a pound of A-grade Humboldt marijuana would fetch anywhere from $2,000 to $4,000, depending on the time and location of the sale.[2] One farmer who made a habit of driving his marijuana to Las Vegas received $5,000 a pound for his efforts. Prices that high made it worthwhile for growers to accept the risk of criminal prosecution or crop confiscation—both risks were accounted for in any responsible grower's business model in those days. But legalization, in California and elsewhere, has brought with it the sobering reality that prices will likely never reach those heights again. Thousands of intrepid growers are jumping headfirst into the Great American Green Rush, hoping to secure a foothold in the industry before federal legalization blows the market wide open.

Elaine has been feeling the impact of these many new farmers (and their crops reaching the market) for several years now. The offers she received for her 2016 harvest were emotionally, not to mention financially, deflating. So she, like many others, embraced the tried-and-true wait-it-out method, hoping prices would rebound in the coming months. She waited, month after month, from the end of the harvest season, through the rainiest winter and spring seasons in Humboldt history, and into the early summer planting season. Prices never budged. Finally, after sitting on her 2016 harvest for nearly a year, she unloaded it for a personal-record-low $1,000 a pound. Not willing to compromise on the quality of her product, Elaine doesn't know if she still fits into the farming industry she's grown up with.

"You know, I just don't know if I have it in me anymore," she told me. "Things are so different now."

The market hasn't been any kinder to Jack, though he fits the mold of a young ganjapreneur who can more nimbly respond to rapid shifts in the market. His sun-grown marijuana still competes with high-end crops, and fetches prices accordingly. But those prices have collectively come down, and he's being forced to diversify. Among his growing list of ambitions: farm through the winter (previously unheard of in Humboldt); launch a commercial clone operation; ramp up hash oil production (to feed the explosive growth of the marijuana edibles market);[3] develop a brand for his marijuana; and, most audaciously perhaps, open a network of dispensaries to sell directly to the consumer. His strength and competitive edge is predominantly botanical, so some of these ventures will require extending himself into less comfortable territory. But the Green Rush is gaining speed, and he intends to keep pace.

In 2017, outdoor growers in the Emerald Triangle of northern California faced an additional threat their indoor competitors did not: wildfire. Fires burned across the Northwest, through parts of Washington, Oregon, Idaho, and California, for months on end, including the crucial weeks of harvest, blanketing the region in smoke. For Jack and other viticulturists, the smoke damage was calamitous—many didn't bother harvesting their grapes at all. Marijuana buds aren't as sensitive to smoke damage as grapes are, but they aren't impervious either. The Emerald Triangle's sustained run of excellence should protect its reputation from a seemingly fluky drop in quality, but promoters of indoor-grown marijuana are sure to point out that the risk of wildfire in the American West is persistent and real, and not likely to disappear.

From a macro perspective, however, the American marijuana farming industry is alive and well. Arcview, an industry analysis firm, estimates that 15 million pounds of marijuana were produced in the United States and Canada in 2016.[4] The value of that production was a staggering $56 billion in revenues.[5] There is little precedent for the annual growth rate that the legal market for marijuana has experienced in recent years. That rate is likely to grow larger still in the coming years, as more states join the legalization movement, and more consumers are introduced to legal marijuana products that meet their needs. The size of the farming community is likely to grow in response to these trends, with increasing numbers of novice farmers producing marijuana exclusively as well as more conventional farmers incorporating marijuana into their crop portfolio. The Big Marijuana barons might be kept in check for a while, waiting for the federal government to unlock the corporate floodgates, but eventually they too will find their way in.

What is frustrating for some of the old-timers, like Elaine, is that it hasn't always been this easy to get in the game. Veterans of the war on drugs made large profits in the prohibition era, but they sacrificed and toiled in hardship to get them. They birthed the American marijuana farming industry and nurtured its youthful development. Like any parent, it can be difficult to watch that baby enter maturity and fly the coop, embedded with and embracing a new group of friends.

Will Elaine and the rest of the marijuana farming pioneers of the twentieth century have a role to play in the new marijuana industry? I believe they will, in part because their inventive identity is central to the entrepreneurial ethic that pervades the Green Rush. And in an effort to create the ideal marijuana industry for the American people (whatever that ideal may be), it would be foolish to ignore the wisdom of our most experienced and battle-hardened marijuana farmers. Most of this book is dedicated to thinking about the future of marijuana farming, but no forward-thinking endeavor makes it far without an appreciation of history. Or, as James

Baldwin implored: "Know from whence you came. If you know whence you came, there are absolutely no limitations to where you can go."[6]

The United States' rich history of farming cannabis in the form of hemp obscures the fact that marijuana farming is, relatively speaking, a very new phenomenon in this country. Whatever marijuana was being consumed in the nineteenth and early twentieth centuries mostly came from Mexico, and was fairly low in quality. Even in the twentieth century, when domestic consumption picked up steam and entered into the popular (counter)culture, domestic production lagged behind considerably until the latter half of the century. The Emerald Triangle's renegade growers launched the American marijuana farming movement in the 1960s and 1970s, but production really took off in the twenty-first century when states started flaunting the federal government by authorizing cultivation and unleashing the power of American agriculture. Ironically, many of the states leading the legalization charge today are the same states that started the prohibition movement a hundred years ago.

Ever since the Spanish introduced hemp to their American colonies in the sixteenth century, cannabis has flourished in Mexico. Hot, dry, and sunny, with remote and rugged mountain valleys, Mexico provides a perfect home for marijuana. By 1900, it could be found growing in the wild, cultivated by peasants, or rolled up into smoking papers and sold in towns. The economic prospects of the average Mexican, however, were less inspiring. Mexico's political economy was suffering from dictatorship, causing a mass exodus into the United States. Migration intensified during the Mexican Revolution in 1910. Migrant laborers found jobs throughout the western and southern United States, from California produce farms to Texas cattle ranches.

As many generations of migrant laborers all over the world had done before them, Mexican immigrants didn't forget to bring their fondness for marijuana with them to their new home. Cultivation was still taking place in Mexico, but marijuana smoking became commonplace anywhere Mexican laborers could be found. And, like many migrant laborers, Mexicans quickly became vilified by white Americans who resented their otherness and willingness to work for low wages. By the early twentieth century, the nexus between drugs and race was a centuries-old strategy of suppression, and so marijuana became an easy target for governments trying to control the Mexican population.

California, which would eventually become the headquarters of the marijuana legalization movement, was the first state to ban marijuana in 1915. Colorado, Washington, Oregon, and Nevada, among others, followed suit in short order. In Texas, where marijuana was banned in 1919 in a climate of labor unrest, one state senator's rather unscientific observation of the marijuana problem is now legend: "All Mexicans are crazy, and this stuff is what makes them crazy."[7]

Within twenty years, thirty-three states would have marijuana laws in place. But the federal government was slow to jump on the bandwagon, despite protests from the states that its stance on marijuana was outdated. The U.S. military launched a formal study of the effects of marijuana in the late 1920s when it was discovered that consumption was widespread among American soldiers in the Panama Canal Zone. Like the Indian Hemp Drugs Commission before it, however, the report found marijuana to be fairly innocuous and unworthy of extensive controls.[8]

Marijuana prohibitionists found fertile ground in the 1930s. With alcohol prohibition overturned, the temperance movement zeroed in on new intoxicants. By now marijuana was being commonly used in both the Mexican and African-American communities. The drug was especially popular in jazz circles, which raised its profile during the alcohol prohibition era of the 1920s.[9] The rise in popularity caught the attention of federal authorities.

Various federal agencies had asserted some jurisdiction over narcotics during the alcohol prohibition era. But whether due to the corruption or the ineptitude of these agencies, Congress cleaned house in 1930, creating the new Federal Bureau of Narcotics (FBN). Its first commissioner was Henry J. Anslinger, who held the post for thirty-two years and ushered in the federal marijuana prohibition era. Anslinger's longevity in the role is a testament to his skill as a bureaucrat and rhetorician. He had much to gain from a war on marijuana, including notoriety and funding for the FBN. Despite little evidence that marijuana was a social problem on the scale of opium, cocaine, or alcohol, Anslinger whipped the temperance movement into a frenzy. Marijuana users were portrayed in the press as violent killers and rapists, insane degenerates, or innocent children whose lives were shattered after consuming marijuana.[10] Testifying before Congress in 1937, Anslinger declared: "Marijuana is the most violence-causing drug in the history of mankind."[11]

Anslinger was not alone in his quest. He received help from powerful industries that stood to lose if cannabis became a major agricultural product of the United States. Hemp farming was on the verge of a breakthrough in the 1920s, with increasing hope that a decorticator could process hemp fibers on an industrial scale. Some theorized that William Randolph Hearst, who was heavily invested in the timber, paper, and newspaper industries, was using his empire to push anti-marijuana coverage into the mainstream media.[12] Similarly, Lammot Du Pont, head of the petrochemical conglomerate Du Pont Company which invested heavily in plastics and paper-making chemicals, was feared to be lobbying Congress for legislation that could stem the rising tide of cannabis agriculture.[13]

Anslinger and the temperance movement got their wish in 1937, when President Franklin D. Roosevelt signed the Marihuana Tax Act into law.[14] The act did not prohibit marijuana cultivation, sale, or consumption. Instead, it levied a tax of $100 an ounce on each farmer, distributor, retailer, or consumer every time the drug changed hands. Keep in mind: $100 in 1937 had roughly the same buying power that $1,725 had in 2017. At the same rate of taxation, a farmer today would be taxed, on each pound of marijuana, $27,600. The instrument of the Marihuana Tax Act of 1937 was taxation, but the intent (and effect) was prohibition.

At the time the Marihuana Tax Act was passed, marijuana consumed in the United States was still being imported from Mexico.[15] The act did little to address that trend. The act seemed about to deliver a potentially fatal blow to American hemp farmers, but war, once again, revived the industry. When the Philippines fell under enemy control during World War II, the United States lost access to one of the world's largest plant fiber producers. The Department of Agriculture responded with the "Grow Hemp for Victory" campaign, enlisting 20,000 American farmers to cultivate 30,000 acres of cannabis.[16] The campaign was terminated in 1946, and with it the hemp farming industry faded away. But the legacy of the war campaign can be seen across the Midwest today, where wild cannabis still grows around the rural agricultural communities of the American heartland.

The Cold War sustained many of these tensions between drug control and political necessity. On the one hand, Anslinger and the FBN continued to portray marijuana users as an undesirable lot, although now users were characterized as lazy communists, not as violent killers. Marijuana prohibition became a tool for the FBN to fight against communism at home. Anslinger ordered FBN agents to conduct surveillance on scores of high-profile jazz musicians who embodied the counterculture, including Louis

Armstrong, Thelonious Monk, Count Basie, Duke Ellington, and Dizzy Gilles-pie, with the hope of busting them all in one ignominious raid.

On the other hand, the U.S. military agencies had bigger targets than mari-juana; they even sponsored and supported several anti-communist forces that were heavily involved in the drug trade. The CIA and State Depart-ment covertly organized a public relations campaign during the 1950s and 1960s designed to showcase America's commitment to cultural and creative freedom. Those jazz legends that Anslinger was surveilling—including Louis Armstrong and Dizzy Gillespie—represented The American Way to large crowds in Europe, Africa, and Asia throughout the Cold War period.[17]

Jazz musicians may have been the first American marijuana celebrities, but they weren't the last. Jack Kerouac and Allen Ginsberg evoked the spirit of the beat generation's relationship with marijuana through their writing, while Bob Dylan and the Beatles embraced the drug's influence on their music all the way to international superstardom. Marijuana users were no longer perceived to be the violent, unstable ethnic minorities Anslinger wanted the public to believe they were.

By 1963, the majority of people arrested for marijuana violations in California were white.[18] Many users were middle-class college students or graduates. The centuries-old, dependable strategy of associating a drug with a loathsome minority or the lower class wasn't working anymore, as mari-juana had become the drug of choice for baby boomers and young people across the country. One political activist coined the slogan that would come to represent the generation's fierce independence: "Don't trust anyone over thirty."[19] The hippie movement had arrived, and with it an ethic of self-reliance. That ethic would provide the foundation for the rebirth of the American marijuana farm.

Santa Rosa in the early 1970s was a far cry from the growing San Francisco exurb it has become today, as a gateway to Sonoma County's wine region. It was then a small town, populated by a young counterculture generation that found solace in the flower-power ethos of the hippie movement in northern California. Land was fairly cheap then, and the climate as pleasant as it's always been. The intense vitality of San Francisco in the 1960s and 70s was close by if one wanted to jump into the fray. But Santa Rosa was sleepy, more tranquil. It was a safe place for any young hippie to put down roots and still feel a part of the New Left movement.

Elaine came to Santa Rosa during that time to study horticulture at the local junior college. She is a middle child, independent enough to leave home after high school but not so disconnected that she went very far. Her temperament is both strong to the core and outwardly gentle. She doesn't suffer fools easily (hold this thought), but in good company, she giggles a lot.

Elaine wasn't much interested in marijuana in those days, but she loved taking care of plants. She spent her free time outside caring for her garden, poring over her textbooks, or swapping plant care tips with friends. Her first exposure to marijuana growing came when her roommate Kent started growing pot outside in the greenhouse they had built in the backyard. Kent, Elaine, and Elaine's boyfriend Bill shared a quaint three-acre property that came with a small house, the greenhouse, an apple orchard, a vegetable garden, and a horse.

Kent didn't harbor ambitions of making it rich off growing weed, but he liked to smoke it, and thought he might as well grow his own supply. To Elaine it was just another plant, and she was more interested in her vegetables than getting into the weed game. She wasn't seduced by the plant more than by any other, but like any passionate gardener, she could appreciate the unique botanical characteristics and cultivation strategies of cannabis.

But she certainly appreciated having a reliable supply too, she told me. "In those days we were smoking a lot of weed and consuming a lot of cocaine. It was great; he was growing it, we didn't have to buy it anymore!"

Their lives weren't all about the drugs. Taking drugs went hand in hand with the New Left's rejection of mainstream culture and with the activism and protests characteristic of California in the early 70s.

"We thought we were going to change the world. Peace, no more war in Vietnam, civil rights was going to be a thing. The whole society was going to change, people were going to just wake up. We were so groovy and loving and kind, everyone would get stoned and love each other. You know, we were just going to change things," Elaine said, laughing.

After graduating from the junior college, Elaine had vague plans to study horticulture at UC Davis. But first she needed to clear her head and get out of town for a while, so she spent a month in Guatemala. It was the first of many foreign adventures she would take in her life, and she still hasn't been able to shake the travel bug. But as all young travelers learn sooner or later, the world doesn't stop spinning when you're away. When Elaine got back to Santa Rosa, her idyllic little farm had a new member. Her boyfriend Bill had found another woman. This being the early 70s, Bill's hope was that the two women wouldn't mind if he dated them both.

Elaine wasn't having it, and while waiting for Bill to make up his mind, she got a call from her ex-boyfriend Matt. He was living up north in a place called Orleans, California. He was growing marijuana, and he wanted her to come help water the plants. Work for me for three months, he told her, and I'll give you $10,000. Why not, Elaine thought. She packed up her things and headed north. The horse came with her. Bill did not.

That first summer Elaine was thrown into the guerrilla growing scene that was typical of California marijuana farms of the 1970s and 80s. Matt was learning the ropes from a grizzled former logger named Hubert, who was the original farming sage of the region. Orleans, their home base in those years, is located on the Klamath River in northern Humboldt County, today a two-hour drive inland from the coast. There are few human settlements in the area, contrasted with thousands of square miles of rugged national forest lands. Hubert's understanding of the logging industry blessed him with a store of knowledge about the area's public forests and the resources they contained. He knew where to find the flat spots, the water, and the gaps in the forest where young plants could catch some sun.

To Elaine, though, the work took some getting used to. Growing marijuana on public lands undetected required stealth, and stealth required hard labor. Establishing a permanent camp with 600 plants was out of the question; human settlements are too easily noticed. Instead, Matt and Elaine would hike in to their plants on foot or on horseback under cover of darkness, setting up the makeshift farm with whatever materials and supplies they could carry in and carry out, including enough food and water to survive for a few days. Then they would go home, bushwhacking their way through a different part of the forest to keep from establishing a permanent trail that the authorities could find and follow directly to the operation.

It was tough work, and many times Elaine was alone in the wilderness. But she loved living in the forest, working with plants. And she was learning quickly. The next summer, Hubert set her up with her own corner of the forest where she could grow on her own. It was an even more remote and inaccessible location than the grow she had shared with Matt the previous summer, so she invited her younger brother, Ethan, to come up and help her out. Ethan was only nineteen and rail-thin, but he could be trusted. It wasn't a tough choice for Ethan—he was working at a gas station when

Elaine came calling. But even with the two of them pulling long arduous hours all summer, they barely made money. The location was too remote, requiring too much time and effort getting there and back undetected.

Winters in northern California tend to be cold and rainy, providing residents with plenty of time to huddle up indoors next to a wood stove and do some reflecting. Elaine knew she enjoyed marijuana farming, but guerrilla growing in the national forest was too ambitious. She had fallen in love with Orleans, so she rented a small place with some property just outside of town. Her third summer, she found a method of guerrilla growing that suited her. She grew on her leased private land, without any help. It was a nifty transition, allowing Elaine to take odd jobs in the community that supplemented her seasonal farming income while appeasing nosy onlookers. Growing at home required a down-scale, of course. Guerrilla growers knew back then that possession was nine-tenths of the law, and a farm consisting of several hundred marijuana plants didn't present much risk if you weren't there when the cops showed up. Hubert taught Elaine not to fret too much about the authorities; if they find the operation and cut the plants down, you can always grow more somewhere else.

While that may have been good advice in the national forest, it didn't hold true once Elaine's name was on the lease of the property she was growing on. She had no choice but to grow fewer plants. But with a smaller crop to take care of, and a much shorter commute to her farm, she had more attention to devote to each plant. She started honing her craft, and the quality of her product improved—by 1970s standards, anyway.

Walk into a marijuana dispensary today, and you're likely to be approached by a salesperson discussing the hundreds of options in front of you in much the same way a sommelier would walk you through a restaurant's wine list. But in the 1970s, consumers weren't as fussy about their marijuana. In part that was due to a lack of knowledge about cannabis strains and the methods of growing them. Marijuana farmers were doing their best with what they had, but the industry as a whole was in need of innovation. Avid growers started thinking outside the box.

In Orleans, change came in the form of a man named Ralph. Ralph was a grower and a bit of a perfectionist. He was frustrated with the low-grade marijuana he and everyone else in Orleans was growing. Rumors were spreading that Americans could find better weed and better seeds if they ventured abroad. In an era that preceded marijuana normalization and the Internet, such a rumor had to be verified personally, so Ralph left Orleans and trekked straight into the Hindu Kush mountains that form a border between Afghanistan and Pakistan. In the high alpine environment where marijuana has been cultivated and growing in the wild for thousands of years, Ralph found what he was looking for: strains of *Cannabis indica* that produced powerful and cerebral highs. He stayed and learned to cultivate marijuana by killing off all the male plants in a crop, leaving behind only females that produced large amounts of buds in hopes of being pollinated.[20] Growing this way would require more effort and attention to detail, but the end result was a product that would blow away the low-quality buds being hawked back home.

Ralph brought the next generation of marijuana cultivation home to Orleans. The seeds were easily brought through in his carry-on—no authorities knew to look for them. Back at home, he gave seeds to growers in the community, including Elaine, and taught them how to grow the new Hindu Kush strains. Ralph ushered in the rise of the high-quality, artisanal marijuana farm in Elaine's corner of Humboldt County.

Ralph wasn't alone in his quest to revolutionize American marijuana farming; he was one of many Americans who returned home from exotic far-flung locales with more than fond memories and a few souvenirs. By the 1960s, the economy had rebounded from World War II and air travel had become affordable to many middle-class Americans for the first time. The younger generation of hippies took advantage. While many traveled to explore foreign cultures and their own spirituality, others recognized an opportunity to bring foreign flavors home to the United States. These travelers and entrepreneurs established what became known as the Hippie Trail, a route that stretched from Morocco to Nepal, with hotspots in between including Turkey, Afghanistan, Pakistan, and India. The trail brought Americans into contact with some of the world's most ancient and prolific marijuana farming regions.

Returnees from the Hippie Trail brought back a number of foreign innovations and cultural products. The New Left's fascination with South Asian cultures introduced or popularized many cultural icons we take for granted today, including beads, prayer flags, yoga, and meditation. Familiarity with psychedelic drugs and their potential for spiritual awakening increased during this time. But for the purposes of our story, it was the introduction of potent *Cannabis indica* strains, and the know-how needed to cultivate them to produce high-quality marijuana, that marked a turning point.

Travelers along the Hippie Trail were introduced to several historically significant marijuana-growing regions. The first may have been Morocco.

Popularized by the Beatniks in the 1950s and 60s, when Jack Kerouac, William Burroughs, and Allen Ginsberg momentarily resided in Tangier, Morocco is relatively close to Spain's southern coast and European markets.[21] With authorities either unable or unwilling to stem the tide of tourists and expatriates smuggling seeds and hash out of the country, local farmers met the increased demand by increasing production. The Moroccan government did its part by turning a blind eye.[22]

The Hippie Trail continued east to Istanbul, Turkey, one of the largest markets for cannabis in the world. Strategically positioned between Europe and the Middle East, Istanbul facilitated trade between Eastern farmers and Western consumers. Further afield, travelers gained access to farmers growing marijuana in the plant's native habitats. Afghanistan and Pakistan, relatively safe at the time, became an operational hub of the trail. The Afghan government welcomed the new business, disseminating fertilizers to farmers growing marijuana in order to solidify the country's place on the Hippie Trail.[23]

With *Cannabis indica* strains and seeds widely available, as well as hash and hash oil ready for transport, some Hippie Trail regulars organized themselves into an international drug-smuggling syndicate known as the Brotherhood of Eternal Love. The Brotherhood purchased cannabis products in Afghanistan and Pakistan for rock-bottom prices, smuggled them into the United States, and distributed them across the country. It was a wildly profitable venture, responsible for financing the Brotherhood's true passion project of bringing LSD to the forefront of American consciousness.[24] As a side bonus, the Brotherhood introduced American farmers to dozens of new strains of marijuana.

India and Nepal were next on the itinerary of the Hippie Trail. From the mountains of Kashmir to the coasts of Goa, throngs of American tourists reveled in Hindu rituals and spiritual practices. The horticulturally inclined took pleasure in seeing marijuana being grown casually in small towns and villages, much as it had been for centuries. In Nepal, the hippies' demand for marijuana was so pronounced that farmers abandoned their subsistence crops in order to grow marijuana instead. At one point the sudden shift briefly created a food shortage.[25] The market was so overtly lucrative for Nepalese farmers that the government started taxing and licensing cultivation in order to share in the windfall. Westerners just couldn't get enough of the high-grade weed being grown along the Hippie Trail.

The introduction of both high-quality indica strains and the know-how to cultivate them marked a turning point in the evolution of American marijuana farming. Until that point, producing marijuana that was comparable in quality to Mexican ditch weed (relatively low quality, that is) meant that American farmers retained only a small portion of the market in the United States. Mexican farmers could and still can produce vast quantities of low-grade marijuana, and the distribution networks of the cartels could (and still can) export it to U.S. markets with ruthless efficiency. As long as American farmers were producing a similarly low-quality product, they would struggle to compete.

But the new strains introduced by enterprising horticulturalists coming home from the Hippie Trail gave American farmers another option: cultivate high-quality strains and compete in the market for mid- and high-end consumers. By the 1970s, that market was becoming robust. Marijuana was being endorsed (in many cases explicitly) by mainstream or counterculture celebrities like Kerouac, Ginsberg, Burroughs, the Beatles, Bob Dylan, Bob Marley, and Hunter S. Thompson. *High Times* magazine emerged as a go-to publication for many of America's 25 million marijuana smokers, bringing to light the multitude of consumer choices on the market. Like many hobby magazines, *High Times* repeatedly ran stories on the newest and best products available, which often meant romanticizing and popularizing the highest-quality, most potent marijuana strains in existence.[26]

Northern California transformed itself to meet this new demand. What had previously been a modest scene driven by the back-to-the-land movement's pride in their self-sufficiency became a full-blown economic hub of the American marijuana farming industry. The region's unique blend of rugged isolation mixed with ideal growing conditions allowed it to scale up production and obtain a foothold in the national market. Most of the marijuana being consumed in the United States was still being imported from Mexico, Jamaica, or Colombia,[27] but growers in the Emerald Triangle began to establish a niche in the high-end market. California and its northern counties developed a reputation for producing the best marijuana.

Eventually, the federal government took notice. President Richard Nixon was no friend of the hippie movement and its Vietnam protesters. Like many politicians and rulers before him, he saw in marijuana the potential for suppression and control. Yet in May 1969, Timothy Leary, perhaps the most prominent LSD advocate in history, successfully persuaded the Supreme Court of the United States that the Marihuana Tax Act of 1937 was unconstitutional, briefly striking down the act and, with it, marijuana prohibition.[28]

Nixon was furious. He had campaigned on a platform of "law and order," promising to eradicate illegal drug use and to take down the unseemly forces behind the drug trade. The Supreme Court's decision dealt that campaign promise a blow only a few months after his inauguration in January 1969. In need of a strong response, Nixon and his advisors targeted Mexico, which remained by any measure the largest supplier of marijuana being consumed in the United States. Though the Mexican government was making nominal efforts to address widespread marijuana cultivation within its borders, the Nixon administration wanted more. On September 21 of that year they launched Operation Intercept, which became known as the largest peacetime search-and-seizure operation in history.

From September 21 to October 10, 1969, thousands of U.S. customs and border patrol agents were planted at every border crossing spanning the 2,000-mile border with Mexico. Their job: to make a thorough search of 100 percent of the vehicles coming into the United States.[29] By creating a border wall via the world's largest traffic jam, the operation plunged the border regions—as well as economic and political relations between the United States and Mexico—into chaos. Gordon Liddy, one of Nixon's advisors who concocted the idea, described the stated purpose of the operation as being to shut down the flow of marijuana coming into the United States. To that end, the operation left much to be desired, as no more marijuana was seized during the operation than average.[30] But Liddy would later admit that the operation's true purpose was more sinister:

> The result was as intended: chaos. We produced a world-class traffic jam....Operation Intercept has been called a failure—but only by those who never knew its objective. It was actually a great success. For diplomatic reasons the true purpose of the exercise was never revealed. Operation Intercept, with its massive economic and social disruption, could be sustained far longer by the United States than by Mexico. It was an exercise in international extortion, pure, simple, and effective, designed to bend Mexico to our will. We figured Mexico could hold out for a month; in fact they caved in after about two weeks and we got what we wanted.[31]

What the administration wanted was threefold. Politically, Nixon wanted a show of force that would substantiate his "law and order" promises and drum up public support for prohibitionist policies. On that front, the reaction was mixed.[32] While some saw the move as decisive and necessary action, others, especially those even remotely involved in bilateral trade with Mexico, saw the operation as an economic and diplomatic albatross.[33]

Administration officials hotly debated the public relations value of the blockade both during and after the operation.[34]

For a time, however, Operation Intercept was successful in achieving its second objective: reducing the supply of marijuana available in the United States, and therefore increasing the price to levels the younger generations couldn't afford. A drought in Mexico in the summer of 1969 hit marijuana farmers hard, such that the usual supply of marijuana coming over the border was already suppressed by the time the operation was launched.[35] Operation Intercept strategically compounded the existing scarcity in two ways: first, the operation was timed to coincide with the annual harvest of most marijuana crops grown outdoors, when the supply of marijuana is at its highest. Second, it made very clear to anyone in Mexico with sizable amounts of marijuana that now was a bad time to move their product. On this point, the operation was a success. Studies found marijuana to be in very short supply across the United States in the aftermath of the operation, with prices doubling or tripling for lower-quality product. *Newsweek* would conclude that the country "lies in the grip of the worst marijuana famine since the weed began its revival."[36]

Of course, the Nixon administration realized that by increasing the price of marijuana, the drug trade would only become more lucrative for suppliers. Mexico still contained vast expanses of remote land capable of supporting a robust marijuana farming industry, and the economic blockade couldn't be continued forever. The United States would need Mexico's help to restrict supply in the long term. This was Operation Intercept's third objective.

The Mexican government was largely blindsided by Operation Intercept and in no mood to help the Nixon administration, but as Liddy boastfully observed, Mexico badly needed trade to resume. On October 10, 1969, the Nixon administration announced that, as a result of negotiations between the United States and Mexico, Operation Intercept would become Operation Cooperation. The Mexican government agreed to cooperate with U.S. federal agencies in an ongoing effort to eradicate marijuana being cultivated in and exported from Mexico. In exchange, the United States would supply Mexico with weapons, crop-spraying aircraft, and financial and technical assistance.[37] The flow of marijuana resumed shortly after the termination of Operation Intercept, of course, and the administration knew it would have to address the demand side of the equation at some point. But Operation Cooperation, in some small way, set the stage for an alliance with Mexico in the war on drugs.

One year later, the Nixon administration and its allies in Congress successfully reinstated marijuana prohibition. The Controlled Substances Act of 1970 (CSA) was swiftly ratified in response to the Supreme Court's decision to strike down the Marihuana Tax Act. Under the CSA, marijuana was classified as a Schedule I narcotic, a designation given to only the most dangerous drugs that were considered the least useful to society.[38] The CSA gave the Nixon administration the broad powers it needed to launch and sustain the war on drugs abroad and on domestic soil. In time, Congress would use the CSA as the legal foundation to transform the Drug Enforcement Administration (DEA) into one of the most powerful and punitive arms of the federal government.[39] The DEA's powers would quickly include the ability to confiscate property, freeze assets, intercept communications, search without warrants, and gather intelligence on virtually anyone it felt like observing.[40]

The ramifications of Nixon's focus on the Mexican drug trade were felt throughout Mexico. By increasing the risk (and therefore the cost) of participating in the drug trade, Nixon indirectly helped the Mexican marijuana industry to consolidate. What had previously been a market welcoming to small-scale farmers and smugglers was increasingly only possible for a small number of well-organized, well-funded, well-armed international drug cartels.[41] Nixon's successor, Gerald Ford, did not share his absolutist views on the drug trade, and favored a more holistic approach to drug abuse in the United States. But the cartels were beginning to encourage opium production in the traditionally marijuana-producing Sierra Madre mountains of Mexico. When the Mexicans came to President Ford for help, he authorized a multimillion-dollar DEA program designed to eradicate the farms by spraying them from above with an herbicide called paraquat.

Paraquat, unfortunately, was a poor choice. As an herbicide it is nonspecific, meaning it kills every plant it comes into contact with in a matter of hours. It is also toxic—harmful to wildlife, livestock, and, crucially, humans. Exposure to high doses can lead to fatal respiratory and kidney failures. Paraquat has been linked to Parkinson's disease,[42] and continues to be used as a poison in suicides and homicides.[43] It is, in short, a nasty and highly hazardous herbicide that warrants using only in a highly controlled manner.

Unfortunately for the DEA and the marijuana-consuming public, the cartels were in control of the farms being sprayed, and their bottom line has always been more important to them than the welfare of their consumers.

As soon as a crop was sprayed with paraquat, they harvested the marijuana and shipped it across the border to recoup their losses. According to a government study at the time, 13 percent of marijuana being sold in the United States was contaminated with paraquat. If smoked, it was found to cause permanent lung damage.[44] President Jimmy Carter terminated the paraquat program with the hope of reducing the public's exposure, but the Mexican government easily found other suppliers of the herbicide and continued spraying it throughout the Sierra Madre. The cartels, in turn, continued harvesting and shipping the toxic marijuana across the border.

America's focus on the Mexican marijuana industry was felt outside of Mexico as well. With the Mexican supply under constant threat and surveillance, other agricultural regions stepped in to fill the void. Higher-quality marijuana was coming in from Jamaica, Thailand, and, increasingly, Colombia. Made possible by a largely agrarian labor class and a government willing to turn a blind eye because of the marijuana industry's massive profits, marijuana agriculture in Colombia exploded. By 1980, Colombia cultivated more marijuana than any other country in the world.[45] Colombian smugglers used their networks to get the product into the United States, usually through Florida. Some of those smuggling operations used their profits from marijuana to expand into the cocaine trade, becoming, eventually, the world's most notorious drug cartels.[46]

At the same time, American farmers were increasing their share of the market.[47] Though Congress authorized the DEA to engage in law enforcement and drug interdiction on U.S. soil, Mexico had been the focus of Nixon's administration, and Colombia did its part to share the limelight. No one realized how much marijuana was being grown on domestic soil until 1982, when the amount of American-grown marijuana seized by law enforcement authorities was 38 percent higher than the total amount of marijuana the federal government had estimated was being grown domestically.[48] Whatever the true acreage was, it was clear the DEA had grossly underestimated the size of the American marijuana farming industry.

Enter Ronald Reagan, the fortieth president of the United States. Reagan's war on drugs was conducted with a fervor that put Richard Nixon's gimmicky Operation Intercept to shame. The Reagan administration's influence (bolstered by a willing Congress) over minimum sentencing and the consequent rise in prison populations nationwide are now legend. Less well known is the reign of terror he inflicted on American farmers.

The Posse Comitatus Act, enacted in 1878, prohibits the U.S. government from using its military personnel to enforce civilian laws. In effect, the 1878 law protects American citizens from U.S. armed forces. In 1981, Reagan proposed, and Congress passed, the Military Cooperation with Civilian Law Enforcement Agencies Act. This act authorizes the president to employ the armed forces to participate in the war on drugs on domestic soil. Reagan took full advantage, and marijuana farmers were firmly in his crosshairs.

Reagan set the tone by employing a by-any-means-necessary approach to marijuana eradication. His administration was not as hesitant to incur collateral damage as his predecessors had been. Reagan authorized the DEA to spray paraquat (still as toxic as it was in the 1970s) on marijuana crops, even those being grown on U.S. soil. When the plan was blocked in federal court out of concern for the impact paraquat would have on public lands (the DEA wanted to spray guerrilla grows located in national forests in Georgia and Kentucky), the DEA announced plans to use the herbicide on marijuana crops found on private lands instead.[49]

Throughout his presidency, Reagan's rhetorical gifts successfully associated the drug trade with violence and social unrest, creating a favorable climate for state and local politicians to accept the president's newly legal power to provide federal military assistance. Reagan started by sending military equipment and personnel to the front lines of the domestic war on drugs. In 1983, he partnered with officials from his home state of California to create the Campaign Against Marijuana Planting (CAMP). Jointly created by the federal DEA and the California Bureau of Narcotics Enforcement, CAMP enlisted the support of dozens of federal, state, and local agencies in the fight against marijuana farming.[50]

CAMP's modus operandi was simple: the feds would provide helicopters, weapons, espionage equipment and intelligence, personnel, and federal funding to the state and local agencies who had the legal authority to go after California farmers. In practice, that usually meant heavily armed CAMP squadrons would fly helicopters just above the tree line during the harvest months of September and October, scanning the landscape for outdoor growing operations. When they spotted one, the helicopter would land on the property, allowing the CAMP team to cut down and seize all the plants, and arrest any nearby occupants of the property. CAMP's tactics were legally problematic—helicopters would often land on a property without obtaining or providing a search warrant, and unlucky farmers who happened to be with their plants during a raid were rarely read their rights when being detained.[51]

By 1983, the Emerald Triangle counties of Humboldt, Trinity, and Mendocino constituted the most concentrated marijuana farming region in the United States. And for most of its existence,[52] CAMP was firmly focused on the Emerald Triangle and its burgeoning farming industry. Between 1984 and 1995, over 60 percent of plants eradicated by CAMP were located in Humboldt and Mendocino counties alone.[53] CAMP's intentions in the Emerald Triangle went beyond eradicating marijuana plants, however; they wanted to eradicate the whole community. One CAMP commander admitted, "we're going after the community support system that makes it appear as a viable and legitimate enterprise."[54] In the culture wars of the 1980s, cutting down plants wasn't enough: the holy grail was the systematic destruction of the American marijuana farming industry.

CAMP largely succeeded in breeding a climate of insecurity and secrecy in the Emerald Triangle. Some members of the back-to-the-land generation of marijuana farmers left entirely. Many of those who stayed suffered the terrors of militarized helicopter raids as an accepted fact of life. But if CAMP's purpose was to destroy the California marijuana farming community and their crops, it failed on both counts.

Geographically, CAMP's focus on the Emerald Triangle pushed the community to expand into less scrutinized lands. Tactically, many farmers transitioned to indoor agriculture because it was harder for the authorities to spot plants from above or obtain legal permission to enter the premises. It has always been difficult to accurately calculate production figures on the black market, but rough estimates suggest that the Emerald Triangle adapted to the CAMP presence rather well.

When CAMP was established in 1983, California farmers were responsible for growing roughly 15 percent of the marijuana consumed in the United States.[55] By the end of its tenure thirty years later, that share had risen to an astonishing 79 percent.[56] By raising the stakes, CAMP had ensured the price of marijuana would remain high,[57] and resilient marijuana farmers did their part to make sure the supply kept coming.

As for the marijuana farming community and its support system, CAMP made it bend, but couldn't make it break. In fact, the persistent threat of an organized task force of federal, state, and local authorities may have inadvertently strengthened the bonds of the farming community, which up to this point had consisted largely of independent guerrilla growers who didn't have much need for a support system. CAMP's controversial tactics spawned a number of lawsuits organized by marijuana farmers, as well as the creation of citizen observation groups designed to document CAMP's abusive practices.[58] Radio stations in the Emerald Triangle acted as the loudspeaker for an informal calling tree—when someone saw a helicopter, they would report the location and direction to the radio, which would then broadcast the information across the airwaves. The growth of the American marijuana industry during the 1980s and 90s had attracted new types of marijuana farmers who could have sowed division in the ranks. By providing a common enemy, CAMP may have ensured that the community stuck together and survived.

Despite failing to eradicate the California marijuana farming industry, CAMP's impact on the community—and Reagan's legacy—was profound. What had been a cottage industry of homesteading hippies was transformed into a high-stakes war of attrition. When some farmers left the scene, their void was filled by a new generation willing to take up the mantle. Many long-time farmers stuck it out through the peak years of the war on drugs. But for those who stayed, the war took a heavy toll.

By the time CAMP made its presence felt in Humboldt County, Elaine had established herself as a veteran marijuana grower and a fixture of the local community. It had been over ten years since she first cared for Matt and Hubert's guerrilla grow in the national forest. She was growing quality seedless *Cannabis indica* strains wherever she could find a suitable plot of land. Sometimes she grew on her own private land, other times she grew in the national forest or on someone else's remote undeveloped property. She worked odd jobs to integrate herself into the community and supplement her income: she was a caretaker for a fishing lodge on the Klamath River, a cook for a rafting outfitter, a teacher's aide for the public schools, and for a while she lived with a farming community of Seventh Day Adventists.

Through luck or skill (or both), Elaine managed to avoid arrest. Prior to the CAMP era, marijuana raids had been complaint-driven and staffed by local police. On one occasion, while she was tending to a grow in the woods behind the fishing lodge, the lodge owners stumbled onto her plants. Elaine heard their voices coming, ducked into the brush before they could see her, and fled to a friend's house. That night, under cover of darkness, they went back to the grow, dug up all the plants, and replanted them several miles away. When the sheriff showed up at the lodge the next day, the evidence was gone.

After that, she teamed up with her new boyfriend, Alan, and their friends Alma and Beckett. The four of them started growing on the national forest on a steep plot of land overlooking the Klamath River. During the harvest season, they would bushwhack their marijuana downhill to the river, where a friend with a drift boat would be waiting. The boat would carry the whole crew downriver, along with several large metal boxes full of weed stacked on top of each other. Eventually they'd reach a highway overpass where another friend would be waiting with a car to carry the boxes away. It was a solid operation; the location they'd chosen was so remote and unlikely an agricultural destination that when their boat and its merry band of hippies went drifting by a legion of cops dragging a submerged vehicle out of the river, the only interaction between the parties was a brief exchange of friendly salutations. Elaine laughs when recalling the memory. "We just went floating by, with this boat full of weed."

CAMP, on the other hand, was no laughing matter. The program completely altered the mood of the agricultural community in northern California. "It was really horrible at the time. The helos [helicopters] would fly low, and guys would hang out with semiautomatic weapons. It was like the locals were the enemy. I used to have nightmares," Elaine said. "We'd see the helicopter come out of the mountains, and we wondered which friend it was; whose garden had they found?"

Only one of Elaine's grows was raided by CAMP in those early years, though plenty of her friends were targeted repeatedly. Still, plants weren't the real loss. Many locals who lived through those years point to the psychological toll CAMP inflicted. "I felt we were living in a militarized zone, I really did," Elaine said. "I felt it was an us-against-them mentality. They had no qualms about inflicting harm on people. They were ex-military people; they were relishing it."

By then Elaine had obtained a teaching degree from nearby Humboldt State, commuting between school and farm. As her farming life became more militarized, a quiet teaching career working with kids looked increasingly appealing. Everyone she knew was digging in their heels and preparing for a protracted battle with the authorities. Matt, Hubert, Ethan, Alan, Alma, Beckett; Elaine's innermost circle and closest friends weren't going anywhere.

But Elaine was thirty-seven years old and tired. "By then, I'd had it, I was done," Elaine recalls. "When CAMP hit, I said, 'Fuck it, I'm not going to do this anymore.'"

When a school in Mendocino County offered her a job, she left the marijuana scene behind. Over the next twenty years, she bounced around the world from one teaching gig to another, exploring faraway lands and making new friends in places like Peru, Ecuador, Zimbabwe, Burma, and China. She didn't come back to Humboldt County until 2011. A year later, the state of California withdrew its funding for CAMP, effectively disbanding the program. Now, as she approaches retirement, she looks back on those fateful years and struggles to make sense of CAMP and the war on drugs. "I don't even know why they did it. I think about it today and go, 'Why did they do this?'"

To be fair, not everyone growing marijuana in those days was a well-educated peace-loving back-to-the-land hippie. By the time CAMP had made its mark, the farming community was increasingly composed of black-market entrepreneurs attracted by the price of marijuana, which was being inflated and maintained by the risks CAMP and the DEA presented to anyone involved in the industry. There were, at times, outbreaks of violence.[59] But the farming community maintained a level of peace and stability that is uncharacteristic of the illicit drug trade.[60] Perhaps the original back-to-the-land generation was able to establish a culture of tolerance that filtered through to subsequent generations of farmers. Or maybe the non-addictive nature of marijuana use kept the industry away from the type of dependence-driven crimes other drug trades are susceptible to.

Whatever the cause, the community persisted through the twentieth century's most intense assault on American agriculture. For every Elaine that had had enough of CAMP's tactics, there was an Ethan, an Alan, or a Hubert willing to carry on. In fact, CAMP may have inadvertently laid the foundation for a revitalization of the American family farm. By stamping out the biggest growing operations, authorities ensured that no one entity could obtain a significant share of the agricultural market. The marijuana farming industry of northern California during the 1980s and 1990s was fertile ground for any hard-working small-scale farmer. This much was clear to historian Ray Raphael as early as 1985:

> As the government eradicates the larger, more visible plantations, the less visible and safer enterprises might enjoy a greater share of the market. Governmental

eradication of marijuana agribusiness therefore can serve as a protective subsidy for small, independent growers, doing as much for the cause of democratic capitalism as the Small Business Administration could ever hope to do.[61]

Raphael's prediction would prove prophetic. California claimed its spot at the top of the list of suppliers to the American marijuana market on the backs of the tens of thousands of small-scale farmers willing to risk prosecution by growing marijuana. By some estimates there are now at least 50,000 marijuana farms in the state of California alone.

As the war on drugs era transitioned into the modern era of legalization, many of these farmers continued to adapt. By and large, the market is still dominated by thousands of small farms, instead of a few large conglomerates. But every marijuana farmer now knows the landscape is shifting underneath him or her, without any clarity on what lies ahead. Legalization has transformed the American marijuana farming industry into a rapidly evolving mass of agricultural entrepreneurs. Together they provide the foundation for the most lucrative cash crop in America. The rapid transition from black-market guerrilla grows to the licensed and legal family farms of the twenty-first century has been nothing short of remarkable.

4 The People's Crop

I have consistently opposed the legalization of drugs all my public life and worked hard against them … I hate drugs.
—Bill Clinton, forty-second president of the United States, 1996[1]

I think there's a lot of evidence to argue for the medical marijuana thing. I think there are a lot of unresolved questions. But I think we should leave it to the states. This really is a time when there should be laboratories of democracy because nobody really knows where this is going.
—Bill Clinton, forty-second president of the United States, 2014[2]

There's a woman in Humboldt County who goes by the name of Sunflower.[3] She's a sixty-year-old widow and mother of three, with emotional scars that betray a life of loss and labor. Sunflower has been in the weed game since the heady beginnings of the back-to-the-land movement. She got her start working guerrilla grows on the national forest, saving up enough money to buy a small plot she could live on and use for a small-scale grow. She navigated the murky waters of the first medical marijuana laws. Today she makes a living as the community's unofficial "Clone Lady," selling baby plants to the community's next generation of farmers.

Sunflower has the sort of casual confidence and been-there-done-that attitude that you'd expect from a veteran of the drug wars, but under the surface there's more contrition than pride. She knows what life as a marijuana farmer has done to her kids, her husband, her friends. Sunflower persevered, but her sixty years are more hardened than most.

Entrepreneurs survive by reading and adapting to market changes. Sunflower knows this—it's one of the reasons she's stayed in business all these years. She also knows the marijuana industry is evolving at a more furious pace now than ever before. Sunflower is preparing to do what very few of her peers will even consider: get legal. At sixty, she doesn't see herself staying in the game much longer, maybe only a few more years. When I ask her why she wants to bother with the arduous licensing process that comes with legalization, her reasoning is dead simple: "Because the handcuffs don't fit anymore. I'm old."

It wasn't always that way, of course. In the 1970s, Sunflower was just a seedling when she left home. She enrolled in classes at College of the Redwoods, a small school on the northern California coast, but she lived with a friend in the mountains an hour east of town. To get to class she had to hitchhike, standing by the side of her sparse country road with a hopeful thumb sticking out. When every ride into school brings with it the promise of meeting someone new, education takes on a broader meaning. Hitchhike long enough, and eventually the ride gets twisted, too, taking the passenger down a road they weren't expecting.

Sunflower was thumbing it on the side of the road on a dreary day in the spring of 1978 when a beat-up truck pulled up next to her. A lean, muscular man sat in the driver's seat, offering relief from the rain and a ride into town. Sunflower jumped into the man's truck, and the two of them never stopped riding together. They were married for thirty-four years, becoming parents, friends, and business partners along the way.

Sunflower recounts her marriage to Denny with fondness ("animal magnetism," as she puts it), but hastens to admit that life as a marijuana farmer in the 1980s and 90s was hard on her family. Like most farmers at the time, she was growing on public lands in the early 80s. The work was tough physically, and CAMP added an anxious psychological component. "We'd get flown [over] all the time. You'd hear this *'whap whap whap whap whap,'* and you'd look up, and there they were. We knew to run." CAMP never managed to drive Sunflower out of business, but she admits she paid a heavy price in the resistance. "It took a toll because you never could trust anybody, you know? It took a toll on me, and it took a toll on my kids."

All of Sunflower's children struggled with their parents' career choice at one time or another. Her adopted daughter Jeanine is deaf and often had difficulty in school. When the DARE (Drug Abuse Resistance Education) program, which teaches kids to stay away from drugs, came to her class, Jeanine took it to heart. She told her teachers her parents were growing marijuana at home, in what Sunflower thinks was an act of teenage rebellion. Jeanine's statement was all the ammunition that law enforcement needed to get a warrant to search the property. Sunflower remembers that day well. "They came busting into our house, and when they took her dad away, [Jeanine] said 'No! No! That's the wrong one. Take her!'"

Sunflower and Denny were both convicted of felonies, and Denny spent time in prison. A couple of years later, their attorney worked out a deal to reduce their sentences. In exchange for $10,000 in cash, a local judge bumped their felonies down to misdemeanors, and expunged the misdemeanors from their record.

But their children's peace of mind couldn't be bought so easily. Sunflower's youngest boy has grown resentful of authority figures, and today he struggles with substance abuse. Her eldest—Denny's son from another marriage—fared better, if for no other reason than he left home before it could affect him too much. When the family was raided, Denny's son was getting ready to enlist in the armed forces. The police searched for him, hoping he would testify against his parents, but Sunflower kept him hidden long enough to see him off to boot camp. "We hid him for a little while, until he could get on with his little life and not be dragged down by his dope-growing parents," Sunflower recalls.

That was only the first raid Sunflower and Denny experienced. Legally it wasn't a very complicated situation—marijuana growing was illegal under federal and state law. But she says the two of them have been raided twice since then, and both raids took place after California voters passed Proposition 215, the Compassionate Use Act of 1996, legalizing the medicinal use of marijuana in the state. Prop 215 didn't say much about marijuana agriculture; it didn't clarify who could grow marijuana plants, how many plants they could grow, or how they could grow them.

Sunflower and Denny thought they were in compliance with Prop 215 when they were busted the second time, but it's still anyone's guess. The two of them were growing a couple dozen plants on their own private property. A police helicopter spotted the plants from the air, and a convoy of vehicles carried out the raid. Sunflower was handcuffed to the front porch most of the day while the police searched the house and took the plants, until finally they let her out of the handcuffs, gave her a ticket, and left.

This time the legal proceedings weren't as straightforward. The district attorney didn't know what to do with the case, so after a year and a half the state dropped the charges against Sunflower altogether. And in a brazen move that demonstrates just how strange the laws surrounding marijuana were at the time, Sunflower sued the state, demanding they return her marijuana. She and her lawyer were confident she would win the case, but shortly after they filed suit the U.S. Supreme Court rendered its decision in *Gonzales v. Raich* in 2005, ruling that the federal government could impose criminal penalties on marijuana growers even in states with medical marijuana laws.

The state of California agreed to return three pounds of marijuana to Sunflower, but she would have to show up in court to receive it. Her lawyer was nervous—the state couldn't guarantee that federal officials wouldn't immediately seize the marijuana and arrest Sunflower as soon as she took possession from the state. But she showed up anyway, scared to death, and accepted the marijuana in open court in front of law enforcement, public observers, and convicted felons wearing orange jumpsuits. The feds never showed up. Sunflower's lawyer couldn't control his excitement, and tried to talk her into going to the courthouse restaurant to show off the marijuana to his colleagues. "Hell no," she said. "I'm going home."

Sunflower believes her audacious victory made her a target for Raid #3. On a hot summer day, she got a call from a neighbor up the road that a convoy was coming her way. This time it was a CAMP unit, and they brought the thunder. A dozen vehicles showed up in her driveway, armed men fanning out in every direction, just as a helicopter was landing next to her house. A plane circled overhead for good measure. Sunflower remembers this group as being "weird." They slit her carport open with knives (for no apparent reason), gathered some household items into a pile, and took turns defecating onto the pile (also for no apparent reason). "Wait wait wait, they just took a shit on your property?" I asked. "Right!" she responded. "They dumped everything right into the middle of the living room, and shit on it. Like, human shit. Piss."

In between excretions, the CAMP unit managed to find four pounds of marijuana. The Prop 215 laws were still vague, but four pounds was enough for the state to charge someone with a felony. A year after the raid Sunflower and Denny received their charges in a letter to their attorney offering to charge one spouse with a misdemeanor if the other spouse agreed to plead guilty to a felony. They accepted the deal, and since Denny was on parole at the time, Sunflower took the felony.

The story took another turn from there. A few years prior to the raid, California voters had passed Proposition 36, the Substance Abuse and Crime

Prevention Act of 2000. Prop 36 allows certain nonviolent drug felons to reduce their sentences after a probationary period. So, Sunflower spent a year on probation before her sentence was reduced to a misdemeanor and expunged from her record.

For a career marijuana farmer with three police raids under her belt (not including raids of her trespass grows on public land), Sunflower's two misdemeanors don't make for an extensive rap sheet. The indirect costs of the raids were a bit more substantial, including attorney's fees, a bribe, confiscated marijuana, and property damage. Still, it could have been much worse. California's ambiguous marijuana cultivation laws may have unwittingly pressed Sunflower out of compliance, but at the end of the day, she navigated the legal system well enough to avoid jail time.

That's the good news. The bad news is that the early days of marijuana legalization placed a veil of uncertainty over the farming community. Even on private lands, no one ever knew if they were farming legally or not. After a while, this relentless tension and anxiety—not to mention the many years farmers spent in court defending themselves—wore people down. Sunflower and her family understand this all too well. "I chose a pretty hard path in life," Sunflower tells me. When I ask her if she would go back and do anything differently if she could, she laughs. "Yeah. Not stuck my thumb out."

By the time you're reading this, the end of marijuana prohibition might seem like a foregone conclusion, if not a reality. California set the stage for the first wave of legalization initiatives when it became the first state to legalize medical marijuana use in 1996.[4] Colorado and Washington broke through the next barrier, becoming the first states to legalize recreational marijuana use in 2012, when Colorado voters passed Amendment 64: The Regulate Marijuana Like Alcohol Act, and Washington voters passed Washington Initiative 502.[5] Since then the pace of legalization has only gained momentum. Following the 2016 elections, medical marijuana use was legal in twenty-nine states, while eight states (plus the District of Columbia) had legalized recreational marijuana.[6] By the end of 2017, only three states maintained a strict prohibition policy on marijuana cultivation, distribution, sale, or consumption.[7] Yet these states represent less than 2 percent of the U.S. population.[8]

There may be light at the end of the prohibition tunnel, but the darkness has not been easy to navigate. Some farmers, distributors, retailers, and consumers have been busted, others have not. Government officials have put regulations in place to address some issues, while entire sectors (e.g., agriculture) are ignored. And on a basic level, there still isn't a clear answer to that most elusive of questions—"Is any of this really legal?"

Speaking generally here, the legalization process in the United States has been messy for two main reasons. The first is that marijuana remains a controlled substance under federal law (the Controlled Substances Act). The U.S. Constitution empowers the federal government to regulate or prohibit marijuana, and the Supreme Court has established that the jurisdiction of the federal marijuana prohibition extends to marijuana grown and consumed wholly within a state's borders. So federal officials can still prosecute anyone violating federal law, even if that person is operating legally under state law.

But prohibition laws aren't self-enforcing. The federal government bears the burden of enforcing federal laws, and in states that have legalized marijuana, the feds aren't getting any help. The marijuana industry is simply too large for the federal government to enforce prohibition on its own. As a result, federal enforcement is inconsistent.

At times, Congress has also withdrawn the Department of Justice's budget to pursue medical marijuana prosecutions.[9] And the extent to which the federal government prioritizes marijuana prohibition is dependent on which politicians happen to be controlling the levers of power. The Department of Justice might take a position on marijuana prohibition under one attorney general that is then reversed under the next attorney general. Or one federal agency may take a position that is inconsistent with the position of another federal agency. Thus, while it is clear that marijuana remains illegal under federal law, the way this basic prohibition plays out can be maddeningly unpredictable.

The second reason the legalization process has been messy is that it is being driven not by policymakers but by organized legalization advocates and by voters—the people themselves. All across the country, medical or recreational marijuana is being legalized at the ballot box by voter initiatives that were proposed, funded, and approved without the assistance of state legislators or governors.

The marijuana legalization movement represents an emphatic rebuke of the typical avenues of policy reform. Politicians remain skittish on the issue of marijuana; many seem to be having a hard time letting go of the law-and-order rhetoric of the war on drugs. But most Americans recognize that marijuana isn't the "most dangerous drug in the United States," as President Reagan claimed it was.[10] And most Americans aren't willing to wait for politicians to make the same realization. According to a 2017 poll, nearly two-thirds of Americans believe marijuana should be legal. Support for medical marijuana is even higher, predictably—88 percent of Americans support legalizing marijuana for medical use.[11] These figures aren't surprising given the wave of victories marijuana legalization initiatives are enjoying at the ballot box. Whether politicians are ready or not, legalization is coming.

While politicians typically see where the winds of change are heading and pivot accordingly, that isn't happening for the marijuana industry, or at least not to a great extent. Most politicians appear content to let voters take the initiative, and offer lukewarm or opportunistic support for legalization after the fact. That isn't a problem on its own, and it's a blessing for legalization proponents that laws can be changed via ballot initiatives in the first place. But this trend has one major downside: policymakers are not prepared to regulate the marijuana industry.

If policy reforms are initiated and enacted in the legislature, the reforms tend to be vetted and negotiated by interest groups, policy experts, and the legislators themselves. Often the policies receive input from the executive branch and the administrative agencies that will be tasked with carrying out the reforms. But a ballot initiative circumvents these processes for better and for worse. Unfortunately, the "for worse" part of that equation is that the government often lacks familiarity with the topic, and doesn't have any specific regulations in place to carry out the voters' intent. As a result, states have to scramble to put meat on the bones of ballot initiatives. In theory, policymakers could start developing prospective regulations in anticipation of a successful ballot initiative; but in practice, they rarely have the foresight or motivation to do so.

To be fair, it's not easy to come up with a regulatory framework for a billion-dollar industry that is being legalized overnight. There are hundreds if not thousands of questions regulators and policymakers must address when crafting their policies. Since marijuana prohibition was put in place in the 1930s, no one in power today has any experience to fall back on—and even if they did, much has changed since the 1930s. The marijuana industry has experienced exponential growth, as has the size and scope of most executive branch agencies. Both the regulators and the regulated are navigating legalization issues for the first time. So yes, of course it's messy.

In 1932, U.S. Supreme Court Justice Louis Brandeis wrote in *New State Ice Co. v. Liebmann*: "It is one of the happy incidents of the federal system that a single courageous State may, if its citizens choose, serve as a laboratory; and try novel social and economic experiments without risk to the rest of the country."[12] From this passage the concept of states as "laboratories of democracy" emerged. Justice Brandeis may not have intended for this concept to be applied to novel social and economic experiments that blatantly flout federal law, but, nevertheless, states have never been more experimental than they are now with marijuana regulations.

Generally speaking, there have been three phases of marijuana legalization. The first phase was launched when Oregon became the first state to decriminalize possession of small amounts of marijuana in 1973.[13] Decriminalization renders minor possession a ticketable offense, instead of a crime. Several states followed suit in the next ten years, but since decriminalization laws typically stop short of authorizing cultivation, distribution, or retail sale, this first phase did not include any meaningful attempts at regulation.

The second phase consisted of the passage of medical marijuana initiatives, which launched the legalization movement in earnest. California was the first to legalize medical marijuana in 1996, and within four years Oregon, Washington, Alaska, Maine, Hawaii, Nevada, and Colorado had done the same. By 2012, Montana, Vermont, New Mexico, Michigan, New Jersey, Arizona, and Massachusetts had joined them.

The third phase represents the maturation of the marijuana industry and its inauguration into legal markets. In 2012, Colorado and Washington became the first states to legalize the recreational adult use of marijuana. They were followed by Oregon, Alaska, and the District of Columbia in 2014, California, Nevada, Maine, and Massachusetts in 2016, and Vermont in 2017. This third phase is ongoing, and includes more and more decriminalization and medical marijuana legalization initiatives every year. By the time you're reading this paragraph, it will likely be out of date.

One might think the California model would have set a precedent for other states to follow, since the state legalized medical marijuana in 1996, years before legalization was viable in other states. But California's Compassionate Use Act (CUA) was sparse, and the legislature barely raised a finger to flesh it out with statutory or regulatory amendments. Thus, the California model wasn't much of a model at all. This is doubly true with respect to agricultural regulations. While California made some attempt to regulate the retail and consumption side of the supply chain, the agricultural sector barely registered. The CUA, for example, did not assign regulatory authority to an administrative agency, articulate limits on possession or cultivation, or propose a broad regulatory framework within which the state or local governments could operate.

In the wake of the CUA, a legal medical marijuana industry was created in California, and the industry experienced tremendous growth,[14] notwithstanding the absence of any meaningful state regulations. The CUA's shortcomings eventually prompted the state legislature to enact the Medical Marijuana Program Act (MMPA) in 2003, which, among other measures, restricted the number of plants medical marijuana patients or designated caregivers could cultivate,[15] and assigned further regulatory authority to the attorney general.[16] Even these limits, however, became legally ambiguous guidelines after the California Supreme Court ruled that the rights established by constitutional amendment Proposition 215 could not be limited by legislative act.[17] So the upshot of these early experiments with marijuana legalization is that California's burgeoning marijuana industry went more or less unregulated for twenty years.

In the absence of regulation, marijuana cultivation in California exploded, with approximately 50,000 marijuana farms accounting for 60 percent of all marijuana grown in the United States by 2015.[18] Today there are as many marijuana farms in Humboldt County as there are wineries statewide.[19] This unchecked growth in marijuana agriculture had consequences for the sustainability and potential growth of the industry. The environmental impacts of marijuana farming were also coming to light, and as the prospect of full-blown recreational marijuana legalization was nearing reality, the state was conspicuously unprepared.

Fortunately, the looming 2016 ballot initiative lit a fire under the legislature. In January 2016, the Medical Marijuana Regulation and Safety Act (MMRSA) came into effect, with ambitious proposals to create comprehensive regulations for marijuana agriculture.[20] The MMRSA assigns authority for various regulatory responsibilities to a variety of state agencies, including the Department of Food and Agriculture, Department of Fish and Wildlife, Department of Public Health, and the State Water Resources Control

Board.[21] As the author of the bill put it: "Cultivators are going to have to comply with the same kinds of regulations that typical farmers do ... [marijuana is] going to be treated like an agriculture product."[22]

It took twenty years to get there, but marijuana cultivation was finally recognized as an agricultural activity in California, and is now starting to be regulated as such. When California voters legalized recreational marijuana use with Proposition 64—the Adult Use of Marijuana Act (AUMA) of 2016—the MMRSA's basic framework was incorporated into the new law. Though California wasn't fully prepared for recreational legalization, the state's policymakers, administrative agencies, and regulated farmers at least had some notice of what was to come.

The first states to legalize recreational marijuana use didn't do much better with agricultural regulations, though they did try to address the issue. In Colorado, for example, a task force established to investigate legal and regulatory issues and to propose legislative and executive actions appropriately identified some agricultural issues,[23] such as the need to regulate pesticides and waste products, to tax cultivators, and to establish cultivation limits,[24] but broader issues central to agricultural development (such as water use or permitted cultivation practices) were not addressed.[25] Colorado assumes that marijuana cultivation will take place indoors for the most part, and has set up its regulatory framework accordingly.

Washington's Initiative 502 authorized the State Liquor Control Board to enact cultivation regulations,[26] but otherwise lacked depth in its treatment of agricultural issues. According to some in the Washington marijuana farming community, Initiative 502 may have been drafted to prioritize civil liberties and sentencing reform, while the future of the agricultural sector of the marijuana industry was less of a concern. Notably, Washington permits marijuana cultivation only by commercial farming operations; personal home grows are prohibited.

Some states are belatedly addressing the agricultural dimension of the marijuana industry, but attempts are often half-hearted, thus stunting the farming community's development. In some cases, states have considered regulations that would limit marijuana farming to a select group of large-scale operators. Though these consolidation-by-design proposals would not allow a small-scale marijuana farming culture to take root, they do offer a significant advantage to regulators: by limiting the number of legal cultivators, states can more easily monitor the industry and enforce regulations. For example, while California struggles to regulate tens of thousands of marijuana farms, states like Florida[27] and New York[28] limit cultivation licenses to less than a dozen. This approach allows the state to carefully select responsible farming operations, makes it easy to monitor cultivation, and buys time before presumably shifting to a more expansive model. With so few farmers, states can lavish regulatory attention on the licensees to ensure compliance, or craft site-specific rules depending on the needs and cultivation infrastructure of the operation.[29] And in a sense the system is predictable by making it clear that only a select number of businesses may cultivate marijuana.

There are two major drawbacks to this model. Although limiting cultivation licenses might reduce the state's regulatory burden, it is hard to find equity or public support when the state permits only a small handful of cultivators to participate in the market. As an example, Ohio's 2015 initiative to legalize marijuana included a list of landowners who would have had exclusive rights to cultivate marijuana in the state.[30] The attempt to control the market prompted some legislators to introduce a constitutional amendment that would prohibit the state's constitution from being used to create economic monopolies.[31] Voters then rejected the legalization monopoly initiative (which lacked support from some pro-legalization groups) while approving the anti-monopoly amendment.[32]

Even if a state transitions to a more permissive model eventually, the previously licensed farmers will have a government-given advantage over the competition. And while the state may have developed the capacity to create site-specific regulations under the restrictive model, those capacities would be less relevant when cultivation proliferates and a more comprehensive regulatory approach is needed.

More importantly, perhaps, severe limitations on cultivation licenses ignore the existence and persistence of the black market. If marijuana farming were not occurring to begin with or were unlikely to take root, a limited licensing approach might be sensible. But marijuana is widely available in part because domestic cultivation is increasing across the United States, particularly on private lands.[33] With legalization efforts gaining momentum and spreading knowledge on farming methods, marijuana agriculture is unlikely to remain dormant for long. Considering the size and growth of the marijuana industry, eradication of unlicensed marijuana cultivators is also unlikely.[34] Limiting cultivation to a small handful of businesses offers transitional benefits, but is unlikely to be a sound long-term solution.

Surprisingly, perhaps, there has been some promising leadership on the issue at the local level. While it may be easy for state politicians to overlook the fact that marijuana is a crop that needs to be farmed in order to make its way to consumers, county and city governments can't ignore the realities of marijuana farming. In areas where marijuana is being cultivated on a commercial scale, it will likely have an impact on land use patterns, real estate markets and property values, natural resources, tourism, and employment. It makes sense that local governments would be proactive in creating regulations that allow the marijuana industry to grow in ways that are beneficial and acceptable to their local community.

Giving local governments the freedom to experiment makes sense for state officials as well. States may want to foster a multitude of regulatory approaches in order to identify which rules and regulations work best on the state level.[35] In addition, since legalization has thus far taken place primarily by ballot initiative, legislatures may be hesitant to embrace the marijuana industry for political reasons, and providing a strong role for local governments may be an effective way to reduce these political conflicts.

In any case, local governments are likely to use their ordinance power to regulate marijuana agriculture. Ordinances have the force of law, and can be created to regulate a variety of local issues, such as public health and safety, land use, and use of public spaces. Counties or municipalities are granted the power to enact ordinances from state constitutions or state statutes.

The California MMRSA, for example, authorizes local governments to enact local laws in accordance with the state statute.[36] Colorado grants extensive powers to city and county governments, allowing them to increase taxes or prohibit marijuana cultivation altogether.[37] Washington did not initially grant cities and counties the power to enact marijuana regulations, but many municipalities took it upon themselves to enact their own regulations anyway.[38] In many of these cases, local ordinances are being used to prohibit marijuana cultivation, sale, or consumption,[39] while in other cases, ordinances have made relatively minor adjustments to state regulations.[40] Thus far, local ordinances have not been utilized as a major tool for the regulation of marijuana agriculture. In that respect, Humboldt County, California, may be the first county in the United States to enact a comprehensive marijuana agriculture ordinance.

When the MMRSA was signed into law in October 2015, an "inadvertent drafting error" in the law appeared to require that local jurisdictions implement marijuana cultivation regulations by March 1, 2016, or else that power would be returned to the state Department of Food and Agriculture.[41] The unintentionally narrow timeframe made it unrealistic for most cities and counties to develop a comprehensive framework for marijuana agriculture regulation. An urgency statute was signed into law in February 2016,[42] eliminating the March 1 deadline, but by that time many local governments had retained their authority by simply banning marijuana cultivation—an outcome that was not the intent of the statute.[43]

Humboldt County, however, had been working diligently to create the most robust marijuana agriculture framework by the March 1 deadline, and it enacted the Commercial Medical Marijuana Land Use Ordinance in late January 2016. In part, Humboldt County was able to meet the deadline because it had been working on its Marijuana Ordinance for several years, in collaboration with marijuana industry groups and farming representatives.[44] Thanks to the close collaboration between local officials and industry representatives, the ordinance drafting process was able to move forward quickly and with political support.

Humboldt County's Marijuana Ordinance itself is relatively comprehensive in scope, addressing farming styles (indoor, outdoor, and mixed), historical use protections and benefits for existing farms, tiered permitting requirements based on zoning classifications, total farm acreage and marijuana cultivation area, water quantity and quality protections, energy use, and farm labor standards. The ordinance addresses many of the issues explored in this book, and the choices those issues present to local governments.

The ordinance represents a clear attempt to regulate marijuana agriculture in a tailored fashion. Marijuana cultivation limits (no more than one acre) indicate a preference for small-scale farming and a rejection of large-scale consolidation models.[45] Demonstration of sufficient water rights and water quality compliance permits are required,[46] and energy used in indoor farms must come from renewable sources or be offset with carbon credits.[47] The ordinance even attempts to create a "Humboldt Artisanal Branding" certification program for small-scale, organic marijuana farms.[48]

The central tension local governments face when regulating marijuana agriculture, particularly in jurisdictions where marijuana is already a primary crop, is between the need to bring farmers out of the shadows and into the regulatory system, on the one hand, and the need to create and enforce regulations that have a meaningful impact on cultivation and the direction and impact of the industry, on the other hand. The Marijuana Ordinance addresses this tension by incentivizing existing farmers to register and participate with the county by providing benefits to those farmers who step forward within 180 days following passage of the ordinance. Those benefits include a larger maximum cultivation area (43,560 square feet, as opposed to a maximum 10,000 square feet for new farms)[49] and a certificate of good standing to use for the priority processing of state permits.[50] In addition, the ordinance incentivizes the retirement and relocation of existing farms located in environmentally sensitive areas by allowing farmers to cultivate an area four times larger in environmentally resilient areas.[51]

It remains to be seen if the certificate of good standing will have meaningful value, but the cultivation area restrictions on new farms (which would include existing farms that chose not to register by the deadline) are significant, and may provide a competitive advantage to existing farmers, who can cultivate an area over four times larger than new farmers. In my conversations with farmers in the county, "to legalize or not to legalize" has been a frequent topic of debate.[52] Considering the isolationist and independent nature of the marijuana farming industry in northern California, the fact that "going legal" is a hot topic of debate is a promising sign for the county.

There are areas in which the Marijuana Ordinance is not well thought out. It is logical to require that marijuana farmers have water rights sufficient to meet their agricultural needs,[53] as well as water use plans and other documents certifying water use,[54] but the ordinance may require water rights holders to agree to forego any water diversions from May 15 to October 31.[55] Instead, marijuana farmers would be required to collect and store water during the rainy season in quantities sufficient for the dry season between May and October. While there is some evidence that water used for purposes of marijuana cultivation may have adverse effects on water resources during periods of low flow,[56] the ordinance's prohibition on dry-season water use as a general rule is unprecedented.[57]

The environmental impacts of this rule are unclear, as well. While wet-season flows are high and waterways can likely support an increase in diversions, ecological processes may depend on these traditionally high flows, and widespread wet-season diversions and water storage may disrupt the wet-season environment.[58] In addition, since irrigation demands are substantial during the dry season, the environmental impact of building large storage tanks on every marijuana farm, necessitating building materials, construction waste, and a storage footprint, may outweigh the benefits intended by the rule. And, of course, if this rule is perceived to be unreasonable by marijuana farmers, they may reject the ordinance and regulatory process as a whole.

Cognizant of its shortcomings and the hurried nature of its drafting, the Marijuana Ordinance contains a flexibility provision that may reassure skeptical farmers that compliance is attainable. If, upon inspection, a marijuana farm does not comply with the requirements of the ordinance, the farmer may nonetheless be granted a provisional license, as well as a two-year window within which to cure the violation.[59] The provision is somewhat generous with respect to the compliance grace period, and may buy county officials and marijuana farming representatives enough time to address problematic aspects of the ordinance and to make amendments prior to enforcement of violations.[60]

North of the border, Canada has kept pace with the U.S. legalization movement, and appears to be near the end of its national marijuana prohibition. But unlike in the United States, where legalization has been driven by voter initiatives on state election ballots, Canadian marijuana legalization has been pushed by the courts.

A Canadian named Terrance Parker, who suffered from epilepsy and frequent seizures, may be responsible for initiating the end of marijuana prohibition in Canada.[61] Parker attempted to control the seizures through surgery and conventional medications, but found that only marijuana was an effective treatment.[62] Not having a legal source of marijuana, Parker grew it himself, and was subsequently charged with violating federal marijuana prohibition laws.[63] His appeal reached the Court of Appeal for Ontario, whose remarkable decision in *Regina v. Parker* deemed the federal prohibition of marijuana unconstitutional on the grounds that prohibiting medical use in cases where it is necessary represents a deprivation of liberty, security, and fundamental justice.[64] The court characterized Canada's experience with marijuana regulation as "an embarrassing history based upon misinformation and racism."[65]

The Canadian government responded to the decision by passing the Medical Marihuana Access Regulations (MMAR) in 2001. Under the MMAR, a patient with a prescription for medical marijuana could either obtain it directly from Health Canada (the agency tasked with administering the MMAR) or cultivate it at home. The system was, predictably, problematic.

In order to meet its statutory obligation to provide medical patients with access to marijuana, Health Canada awarded a $5.7 million contract to a single company—Prairie Plant Systems (PPS)—tasked with cultivating marijuana on the government's behalf. The results were underwhelming.[66]

PPS first proposed to base its farming operations at the bottom of a former zinc and copper mine in Manitoba, where tests had found elevated levels of heavy metal contamination in air, water, and soil samples. The quality of the marijuana grown by PPS was suspect as well. Although Health Canada claimed a THC content level of 10 percent, tests revealed THC levels were consistently lower, and some biological tests found mold and other biological impurities in the marijuana. There was little evidence that Health Canada was testing the marijuana before delivering it to patients, despite charging them a significant retail markup. And to make matters worse for patients, they were given no choice with respect to the marijuana's psychoactive characteristics or potency, strain, or cultivation method.[67]

The results of the MMAR's cultivation regulations were foreseeable. Of the few patients who were approved for medical marijuana use, very few of them obtained their marijuana from the government.[68] Most—over 80 percent—chose to grow their own supply.[69] Patients who purchased Health Canada's marijuana rated the quality of the marijuana received in very low terms, and many attempted to return the product for a refund.[70] From a broader perspective, it is clear that most Canadian marijuana users continued to obtain marijuana from the black market, despite the existence of the MMAR.

Two years later, the Court of Appeal for Ontario found the MMAR insufficient to overcome the deprivations of liberty, security, and fundamental justice created by preventing patients from accessing medical marijuana.[71] Subsequent decisions reinforced this point,[72] including a 2008 decision invalidating the MMAR's provisions severely restricting the supply of marijuana.[73] The opinion noted that while the government may have an interest in regulating the size and number of cultivators, its regulations cannot be so restrictive as to preclude access to medical patients.[74]

Reform of the MMAR came in 2014 with passage of the Marihuana for Medical Purposes Regulations (MMPR).[75] The MMPR broadens the pool of potential medical users by authorizing licensed physicians to prescribe marijuana for conditions they deem appropriate, doing away with the MMAR's limited list of conditions.[76] In addition, the MMPR withdrew the government as a marijuana supplier, and instead tasked Health Canada with licensing and regulating cultivators.[77] Despite these changes, the supply of legal marijuana remains limited, partly due to the low number of licensed cultivators.[78]

While Canada's experience with federal medical marijuana legalization and regulation is mixed, the new Labour Party–controlled government (brought to power in 2015) is moving forward with promises to legalize and regulate marijuana for recreational use.[79] The Task Force on Cannabis Legalization and Regulation's 2016 report calls for an overhaul of the current regulatory framework for medical marijuana, opening the door to small-scale farmers, promoting environmentally sound growing practices (such as outdoor farming), and envisioning a parallel market for hemp production.[80]

In April 2017, the Attorney General and Minister of Justice of Canada introduced to Parliament Bill C-45, also known as the Cannabis Act.[81] The Cannabis Act proposed to federally legalize the cultivation, distribution, sale, and consumption of marijuana for recreational purposes. Its particulars are vague, primarily authorizing federal and provincial administrators to develop and enforce a regulatory framework by July 2018.[82]

Unlike the MMAR and MMPR, which largely centralized marijuana regulations at the federal level, the Cannabis Act envisions a large role for Canadian provinces. This shift may represent a recognition that marijuana federalism such as that in the United States, in which states are developing their own regulations, has more benefits than costs. Provinces will be free to establish their own regulations on marijuana agriculture, meaning stakeholders are likely to see a diversity of regulatory frameworks being developed and enforced in the next several years. As has been the case in the United States, this diversity may prove beneficial to the Canadian government in evaluating the merits of various regulatory approaches.

For now, the ambiguous nature of the Cannabis Act leaves many questions unanswered for the marijuana farming community. Whereas the Task Force report recommended the government streamline the licensing process and wield its powers to promote small-scale, artisanal farms, the Cannabis Act merely authorizes administrators to develop a licensing scheme. Similarly, while the Task Force report recommended the government promote environmentally sustainable farming practices (by, in part, allowing for outdoor agriculture), the Cannabis Act is again silent on this issue. It seems the federal government would prefer, instead, to allow provinces to decide both issues on the provincial level. While politically savvy, this approach seems likely to lead to the creation of several provincial regulatory frameworks that aren't as forward-thinking as the Task Force had hoped.

In the United States, it is too early to declare a front-runner in the race to establish the model for state regulation of marijuana farming, much less a winner. On one end of the spectrum lies California, with its sprawling and fragmented army of small-scale outdoor farmers. On the other end of the spectrum are states like New York and Florida, with artificially small farming communities composed of a handful of indoor farming operations. What each state has in common, however, are the tradeoffs that come with their model of choice. Consider, for example, the question of whether a state should regulate marijuana like any other crop, or create an entirely new regulatory framework from scratch. One of the difficulties states face in making this decision is that there are few crops that share the same biological characteristics or legal history as marijuana.

Treating marijuana like any other legal agricultural product has some advantages. Most states already have extensive regulations in place to address the issues involved, including farm business organizations; commercial transactions; crop insurance; agricultural estate planning; agricultural financing and taxation; product safety, storage, and labeling; agricultural workers and labor standards; land use and areas zoned for agriculture; and environmental challenges such as water use, pesticides, fertilizers, and agricultural runoff.[83]

Some adjustments would need to be made, of course, to integrate marijuana agriculture into these frameworks, especially when state regulations are intimately connected with federal agricultural laws and policies. But it would not be excessively burdensome for state agencies addressing these components of the agriculture industry to make the necessary adjustments upon legalization and regulate marijuana in a similar fashion as other crops. Similarly, a farmer growing several crops will already be accustomed to the rules and regulations he or she must comply with, and it would not be impractical for that farmer to incorporate marijuana into their crop portfolio and resume business as usual.

Perhaps, several years or a few decades from now, marijuana will be regulated like other crops. At least initially, however, as states transition to a legal marijuana market, it seems unlikely that marijuana can be accommodated into existing frameworks without creating significant regulatory disruptions. There does not appear to be sufficient political will in place to legalize marijuana and treat it like other crops. Because so much regulatory atten-tion is being placed on where and how marijuana is sold, purchased, and consumed, regulators have included marijuana cultivation in their tailored regulatory frameworks in order to maintain oversight of the supply chain.[84] While that approach has not induced regulators to consider the full spectrum of agricultural issues presented by marijuana, it has removed marijuana cul-tivation from the usual regulatory process other crops would be subjected to.

In addition, where states have acted to restrict the number of farmers cul-tivating marijuana, or the amount of marijuana that may be cultivated by each farmer, they have done so in part to restrict the size of the legal mari-juana market. This may not be restricting the size of the overall marijuana market (which includes the black market)—and in that respect states may be losing out on tax revenues—but the objective is not without merit. The marijuana industry is large and unwieldy, and regulating the industry with-out help from the federal government is a heavy burden for state agencies. In fact, Colorado's neighboring states have argued to the U.S. Supreme Court that its legal marijuana products have placed undue stress on their own state agencies.[85] It is not unreasonable that states would seek to gradually incorpo-rate marijuana into their regulatory frameworks, and doing so may require tailored regulations that remove it from established agricultural regulations.

Beyond this pragmatic concern, treating marijuana indifferently may not be in the interest of the marijuana industry, or the individual states and their marijuana farming communities. An unrestricted approach may lead to the commoditization of marijuana and the consolidation of marijuana farms. In addition, because marijuana has been a black-market agricultural product for decades, it is not entering legal frameworks looking like a tra-ditional agricultural product. Many marijuana farmers grow their plants indoors, for example, instead of in outdoor fields.[86]

Many existing farmers who have been cultivating marijuana on the black market have not been subjected to any agricultural rules and regula-tions. They may not, for example, have valid water rights, land zoned for agriculture, or a sophisticated understanding of administrative law and the permitting process. Subjecting these farmers to the weight of existing regula-tions overnight is within a state's administrative powers, but that approach may come at the cost of alienating those farmers and discouraging them from participating in the legal system, perpetuating a robust black-market farming community. If states are to incentivize participation by existing marijuana farmers, while creating a framework for marijuana agriculture that is responsive to the best interests of states, farming communities, and the marijuana industry, a gradual transition into existing agricultural frameworks may be needed.

A state's willingness to allow local governments to regulate the marijuana farming community also has some weighty tradeoffs. Several states have embraced a decentralized approach, which certainly has benefits. Distributing power among local agencies engages those agencies in the regulatory process. In doing so, the regulatory framework capitalizes on the localized expertise, heightened awareness of changing conditions, and existing relationships between local stakeholders that collectively form a promising recipe for good governance.[87] Simply put, local actors are knowledgeable about their community and provide legitimacy to local regulations. Conversely, there is often resistance to top-down policies that don't reflect local realities, and this resistance can manifest itself in noncompliance with regulatory requirements.[88] By allowing local agencies to create their own policies or manage their own natural resources, the collective whole develops resilience by experimenting with different strategies or approaches; some of these experiments might fail, but others could foster successful innovations that can be replicated in other jurisdictions.[89]

These general benefits of decentralization are particularly applicable to regulating marijuana agriculture. Marijuana remains a controversial political issue, and its liberalization benefits from allowing legalization opponents to enact policies they are more comfortable with.[90] In regions like northern California where a large cultivation community exists in a remote and unique social setting, local officials are better suited to engage an introverted industry than state or federal officials. They are also more likely to develop regulations that reflect the realities of marijuana cultivation, on the one hand, and the ecological or economic conditions of the region, on the other hand.

The North Coast Water Quality Control Board, for example, has put forth a water quality regulation program for marijuana cultivation that was modified based on feedback from marijuana farmers in the north coast region.[91] The Central Valley Water Quality Control Board did the same in the Central Valley.[92] Both programs are integrated into an interagency, statewide strategy for marijuana irrigation regulation that should facilitate coherence across regions.[93] This type of regulatory structure is especially helpful when states are regulating an industry—like marijuana—that is new or unfamiliar, with few established blueprints for success.

If states pursue a decentralization strategy, however, they will be exposed to certain vulnerabilities. Local agencies and jurisdictions may be authorized to develop and enforce their own regulations, but they may not have the institutional capacity to do so. Regulating marijuana agriculture may involve complex tasks—such as hydrological modeling or drug trafficking enforcement—that local agencies are ill-equipped to handle.[94] Regulation requires investments in human, infrastructural, and technological resources that states may be unable to provide to local agencies, resulting in some jurisdictions with well-funded agency operations and others with little to no regulatory capacities.

A corollary of the institutional capacity challenge is that local agencies may not be equipped to regulate on two dimensions simultaneously, as the marijuana-agriculture nexus requires. Colorado's Marijuana Enforcement Division, for example, is defined by its regulatory identification with marijuana, but is not associated with agriculture.[95] The state's Department of Agriculture, conversely, is equipped to regulate traditional crops but has received little guidance on how to address marijuana cultivation.[96] When the department reached out to the federal Environmental Protection Agency (EPA) for guidance on which general crop group (e.g., herbs, spices, vegetables) marijuana fits into for purposes of pesticide regulation, the EPA could only state that marijuana fits into none of these groups.[97]

Colorado's Marijuana Enforcement Division and Department of Agriculture are both state-level agencies that do not have sufficient interdisciplinary expertise at present. The challenge can be more pronounced at local levels where it can be difficult to establish regulatory capacity on one dimension, much less two.

Efforts to decentralize power away from a central government and toward local governments can also, if hastily or sloppily designed, look more like power abdication (in which governments shift an unwanted burden of regulation onto another jurisdiction) or power fragmentation (in which regulatory authorities are ambiguously spread among many different agencies). Although transferring power from state to local agencies has its benefits, power abdication is a problem because the state retains an important role in supporting and coordinating local initiatives.[98] On the other hand, power fragmentation can also be a problem when it leads to overlapping mandates, uncoordinated regulation, or counterproductive policies.[99]

At the moment, states do not have answers to these structural questions. They are each experimenting with legal marijuana farming for the first time, and it is only natural that there will be setbacks. California's policymakers have been explicit in their goal of trying to create a marijuana farming community that is inclusive and protective of the tens of thousands of small-scale farmers in the state. California Lieutenant Governor Gavin Newsom said that "legalization should not be about replacing one cartel with another."[100]

And yet the California Adult Use of Marijuana Act (AUMA) of 2016 may undermine that goal. While the previous law limited the total canopy size of indoor farms to half an acre, and outdoor farms to one acre, AUMA's drafters included a provision that would allow the state to issue Type 5 licenses. No canopy size limits are imposed on Type 5 licenses, paving the way for large-scale, industrial production of marijuana.[101] Large-scale cultivation may flood the market with cheap marijuana, at the cost of quality control and the livelihoods of the state's many artisanal small-scale farmers.

Type 5 licenses cannot be issued before 2023, so the state will have time to consider the issue. This was, ostensibly, the purpose of the provision—to give the state more regulatory flexibility. When I met with California attorney Richard Miadich, one of the authors of the bill, he told me it was tough to figure out where to set the acreage limits. If the limits were too low, the black market would stay alive. If the limits were too high the market would be flooded with cheap marijuana and prices would drop through the floor. At least this way, regulators would have options.

"We really did want the industry to develop in a way that encouraged small growers and medium-sized growers, and discouraged the Big Tobacco–type entities from coming in and trying to dominate the market," Miadich told me. "My hope would be that we start with small cultivation—I like the idea of preserving the unique culture of certain regions in California. But it's hard not to see some cultivation in areas where there was previously no presence of this industry."

When I asked Miadich about the Type 5 licenses, he insisted state regulators retain the tools to fine-tune acreage limits. "We wanted to ensure that, at all times, regulators be mindful of and guard against monopolization and unfair business practices by large operators," he said. To do that, Miadich and his team made sure regulators considered consolidation and monopolization trends when renewing farming licenses.

Will California's marijuana regulators be mindful of monopolization and unfair business practices when the time comes? AUMA might give them the flexibility to make adjustments over time, which is a strength of the law. But the open-ended nature of the Type 5 license provision adds a dash of uncertainty to the farming community. A battle between small-scale farmers and agricultural conglomerates may loom large on the horizon.

The size of the marijuana farming community in the United States is already substantial, and is expected to grow in response to increases in demand from legal consumers. Legal cannabis spending in the United States and Canada is expected to reach $11 billion in 2018. That figure is expected to rise to $22 billion in 2021.[102] But these numbers aren't close to representing the full picture of marijuana transactions, because most consumer spending in the United States is still taking place on the black market. Even though California has the largest legal market in the country, only a quarter of marijuana sales in the state take place on the legal market; the rest is illicit.

Even at the state and local scale the economic impact of legal marijuana farming is evident. In Washington, cannabis (including hemp and marijuana) became the state's second most lucrative crop in terms of annual sales only four years after recreational marijuana was legalized. The most lucrative crop—apples—uses 148,000 acres of farmland in the state. The third most lucrative crop—wheat—requires 2,215,000 acres of farmland. Cannabis farming uses a measly 411 acres.

Farmers will need to maintain or increase production levels to meet expected increases in demand. In 2021, the legal market will consume 5 million pounds of raw marijuana buds, and yet this will only represent a quarter of the marijuana that will be produced in the U.S. and Canada.[103] Again, most of the marijuana crop produced domestically will be sold on the black market.

Estimates of black-market industries—or in this case, a gray-market industry—are notoriously difficult, with a high potential for variance. But as the marijuana industry matures, market figures start to gain focus. What these best estimates can tell us today is twofold. First, there will continue to be strong demand for marijuana. Since the federal marijuana prohibition is still intent on preventing international or interstate marijuana trade, domestic marijuana farmers are in the best position to capitalize on this increase in demand.

Second, the black market will continue to provide farmers with lucrative opportunities to ignore the legal system. If that is the case, states will need to create regulatory frameworks that incentivize farmer participation. If the only incentive is a legal license, while the compliance costs include byzantine paperwork requirements, onerous taxes and licensing fees, and hyperspecific cultivation requirements, farmers will turn around and walk in the other direction, back to the unregulated confines of the black market.

Sungnome Madrone has been thinking about economic incentives in order to identify some regulatory approaches that might encourage small and medium-scale farmers to come out of the shadows. A hydrology expert at Humboldt State University in northern California, Madrone doesn't think states have found the right balance yet. "It's a very basic economic concept in regulation, no matter what the industry is: carrots are more effective than sticks," he explained. "I strongly support local, small, organic, low-energy-use farms, but how do we get to a place where we have this responsible industry? I think we're going to get there faster by providing incentives for good stewardship." At the moment, those incentives are lacking. "I would suggest the number of financial incentives for small-scale growers is nonexistent; it doesn't pencil out," Madrone tells me. "It doesn't take a genius to realize it's going to cost a fortune for them to come into compliance."[104]

Madrone proposes tax write-offs for marijuana farming expenses that benefit the public trust—investments that reduce a farm's impact on water and energy resources, soil, or wildlife, for example. Or cultivation license renewals could be streamlined or issued to farmers without fees if they agree to environmental audits. Regardless of the approach, it seems likely that states will need to continue to refine their regulatory programs. Sticks may be necessary at times, but black-market farmers need to see some carrots, too. If states want small-scale family farms to survive, they'll need to meet those farmers halfway.

If there's one advantage small-scale farmers have over the large-scale agribusinesses waiting in the wings, it's that the large-scale agribusinesses are still waiting in the wings. Relatively large operations are popping up in legal state markets, but they remain small in the grand scheme of things. Big Marijuana investors know they need to wait for the federal marijuana prohibition to be lifted. Until then, the largest operations will remain the first to be targeted and prosecuted by the feds. In that sense, the unique dynamic of marijuana legalization in the United States—in which the federal government maintains a ban on interstate marijuana trade while discouraging large-scale cultivation—is a sneaky benefit for family farmers. The big players can't play yet, and the interstate commerce ban allows each state to create a farming community that's protected from outside competition.

It's not clear how much longer this cover will last. For now the Trump administration doesn't seem enthusiastic about marijuana legalization. And even if Congress removed marijuana from the Controlled Substances Act, the federal government might still be able to enforce a de facto prohibition pursuant to the Food and Drug Administration's authority to regulate drugs and pharmaceutical products.

Indeed, the federal government does not show any intention of surrendering in the war on drugs. The DEA confiscated 5.3 million domestically grown marijuana plants in 2016, the highest total since 2011. Most of these (over 70 percent) were seized in California. Meanwhile, only 7 percent of confiscated plants were taken from indoor grows.[105] The target is the same as it ever was: California's mammoth outdoor farming community. While the community has grounds to feel persecuted, it may be of some solace that the federal government's relentless and somewhat tone-deaf pursuit of marijuana farmers may be keeping Big Marijuana from becoming the economically disruptive force many fear it will inevitably become.

I, for one, don't think that disruption is inevitable. There will be some mix of small, medium, and large-scale farming operations, to be sure. But there are too many farmers and too many activists interested in creating a small, local, sustainable marijuana farming model for that model to be eliminated from the market completely. Still, if family farmers are going to stick around, they'll need to address some of the most pressing issues facing the farming community: How should local farming regions protect themselves? What should a marijuana farm look like? How can marijuana be cultivated sustainably? And how can marijuana and hemp farmers coexist?

At this moment, there is an unprecedented opportunity for anyone interested in the marijuana industry to help mold it into the shape they want it to take in the future. The rules are being written by policymakers who have never addressed these issues before and don't know how their constituents feel about them. Most of them aren't beholden to Big Marijuana interests (yet). The legalization movement is far from over, but the marijuana industry isn't waiting for the movement to come to a tidy conclusion. The marijuana farms of the future will be shaped by the agricultural policies that farmers and consumers ask for today.

Sungnome Madrone laments the fact that many Americans haven't been engaged in local or state politics, but he sees change on the horizon. "People are waking up," he says. "I'm not some dreamer that thinks there won't be large-scale operations with Philip Morris or whoever. But I do believe people will organize. I see a population across the state and across the nation that is waking up and engaging in their communities in ways they never have before. They will push these issues for family farmers, and I think the power of that will continue to grow."[106]

5 The Power and Potential of Marijuana Genetics

No other human occupation opens so wide a field for the profitable and agreeable combination of labor with cultivated thought, as agriculture. I know of nothing so pleasant to the mind, as the discovery of anything which is at once new and valuable—nothing which so lightens and sweetens toil, as the hopeful pursuit of such discovery. And how vast, and how varied a field is agriculture, for such discovery. The mind, already trained to thought ... cannot fail to find there an exhaustless source of profitable enjoyment.

—Abraham Lincoln, sixteenth president of the United States

The marijuana industry is evolving at a furious pace. Keeping tabs on all the ways in which the industry is evolving, however, is a difficult undertaking. And as the industry evolves in several directions simultaneously, debates flare up between industry stakeholders. One of the less obvious battlegrounds, for example, is the nomenclature of marijuana. As I outlined earlier, I refer to psychoactive cannabis strains as "marijuana," nonpsychoactive fibrous strains as "hemp," and the genus of both, collectively, as "cannabis." Many state legalization statutes similarly refer to psychoactive cannabis as "marijuana," such as the California Adult Use of Marijuana Act. The DEA, for its part, uses the terms "marijuana" and "marihuana" interchangeably.

Recently, while speaking with a farming advocacy group in California, I was asked to stop using the word "marijuana" and start using the word "cannabis" instead. From their perspective, the word "cannabis" sounds more professional, and its use will help legitimize the industry.[1] They may have a point—in Canada, where hemp was already legal, the government proposed a marijuana legalization bill known as the Cannabis Act. Perhaps "cannabis" is a more politically palatable term. When I raised that point with a different advocate, however, she thought it would be offensive to stop using the word "marijuana," in part because the Hispanic origins of the word honor the Hispanic history of the plant's cultivation in North America. Besides, she said, "cannabis" is a terribly imprecise term. If you say "cannabis," are you referring to marijuana, hemp, or both?

In truth, "marijuana" is imprecise too. I use it as a convenient reference to psychoactive cannabis, and many others do the same. But marijuana can be broken down into the *Cannabis* genus's member species: *Cannabis sativa* and *Cannabis indica*.[2] Sativa strains tend to grow tall, skinny plants, with long slender leaves. Native to the tropics, sativas are less dense and therefore less susceptible to mold and mildew. They take a while to flower, but when they do, the yields are robust. Indica strains, on the other hand, grow short and bushy plants, with fat buds. Native to dry mountainous environments, indicas are frost-resistant and quick to flower. When smoked, sativas and indicas produce a different sensation as well. As one grower described it to me, "sativa gets you high, indica gets you stoned."

It is often said that the introduction of *Cannabis indica* to the United States in the 1970s is what allowed the American marijuana farming industry to really take off. Before that, growers were using the seeds they found in their personal supplies of Mexican marijuana. Those tropical sativa seeds weren't as well suited to life north of the border, so the quality remained low. For a few years prior to the introduction of indicas, what was being sold as marijuana in northern California usually consisted of a potpourri of buds, seeds, leaves, and stems. As you might imagine, it wasn't a big money-maker.

When folks like Ralph came back from Asia with *Cannabis indica* strains, the product improved in a few obvious ways. First, knowledge of cultivation methods was spreading. Farmers were learning that by isolating female marijuana plants, they could supercharge the females into growing large, plentiful buds. As a bonus, without any male plants to pollinate the females, the buds produced by females would also be seedless. Second, indica strains are well suited to life in the United States. They are more frost-tolerant, and because they grow short and stout, are more easily concealed from the prying eyes of law enforcement.

But the true revolution in marijuana agriculture didn't occur because indicas are inherently superior to sativas; both have their advantages and disadvantages, and a consumer base that values the highs they produce. The revolution occurred when the farming community learned that marijuana plants could be forced to breed with each other. By pollinating the buds of a female plant with the pollen of a male plant, a hybrid plant is produced that combines the qualities of its parents. With this fact understood, growers started breeding marijuana strains that were half sativa and half indica. The hybrid strains combined the high yields and smooth highs of the sativas with the resilience and potent highs of the indicas.

It doesn't take a high-tech laboratory to breed marijuana plants. One method is to place a male plant in close proximity to a female plant, wait for the male to pollinate the female, and harvest the seeds that emerge from the female's buds. Alternatively, the male pollen can be collected by shaking it off into a bag and then applying the contents of the bag onto a female. Either way, the planted seeds germinate and become hybrids of their parents. This process can be repeated indefinitely by any thoughtful farmer or breeder, each time producing a new hybrid plant. And, in fact, the process has been repeated so many times over the past fifty years that it would be practically impossible to account for the number of strains in existence. Lists of the most prominent and marketed strains have been compiled,[3] but any such list is invariably incomplete and quickly obsolete, omitting the obscure and new strains being created by breeders and growers every day.

In the 1970s and 1980s, breeding was done primarily by farmers who were simply looking for a higher-quality product. And since the industry wasn't as open back then, farmers spent years in isolation breeding their own unique strains of marijuana. Now that the industry has matured, specialty breeders are developing "designer strains" that isolate a single characteristic and breed plants repeatedly in order to bring out that characteristic.

If you're trying to create a strain that produces beautiful rainbow-colored buds, for example, you start with the seeds of your most rainbow-colored female. Of the thirty plants that female produces, one will produce the most beautiful rainbow-colored buds. That plant is then selected for reproduction, followed by her most rainbow-colored-bud-producing offspring, and so on and so forth until you end up with plants that are consistently producing the characteristic you're looking for, in this case beautiful rainbow-colored buds.

Despite the nascent state of the marijuana industry, breeders have already come up with a dizzying array of strains that feature hyperspecific characteristics.[4] For some time now, American breeders have been considered the best in the world.[5] Breeding is so prolific that a niche industry has emerged in order to identify, categorize, and describe the universe of marijuana strains. Leafly, one of the most comprehensive online resources of this kind, allows users to search for strains using filters that include mood (e.g., lift your spirits; stay productive), activity (e.g., stay active; good night's sleep), symptoms (e.g., fatigue; cramps; nausea), flavors (e.g., blueberry; coffee; sage), effects (e.g., giggly; creative; aroused), and conditions (e.g., anxiety; hypertension; migraines). If all that is enough to make your head spin, there's probably a strain to help you with that, too.

Of course, cultivating marijuana doesn't require breeding. In fact, for a farmer, breeding may be counterproductive. Matt, a farmer I met recently, helped me understand this point. He has been growing in Humboldt County for years, with access to some obscure and unique strains that his father and his father's friends have been breeding for several decades. But for the past few growing seasons, Matt has been exclusively growing a strain called OG Kush. OG is a notoriously high-maintenance sativa-indica hybrid, known among farmers as a pain in the neck to grow because of its weak disposition, small buds, and low yields. Most years Matt gets, at best, a couple of pounds of marijuana per plant. Among consumers, though, it's extremely popular, with a knock-you-to-the-ground potency that many of today's marijuana users are looking for. For this reason, Matt has never failed to sell his OG for a good price.

Matt's brother, Jakob, on the other hand, is fully invested in breeding and growing his own strain. Jakob has spent decades perfecting a strain—originally a hybrid created by his father—that is easy to grow and produces massive, fist-sized buds. A single plant of this strain can yield ten pounds of marijuana. Unfortunately, in his quest to create a strain that produced big buds and big yields, Jakob neglected to consider the consumer experience. His marijuana doesn't smoke that well, and potential buyers don't know what to make of the oversized buds. By October 2017, when the market was flooded with that summer's crop of marijuana being harvested all over the country, Jakob still hadn't sold his 2016 harvest.

A more strategic breeding effort, though, can be lucrative for even the smallest-scale farmers. One of Jack's friends, Vinny, complements a modest income from marijuana farming with income from a music promotion business, setting up music festivals up and down the West Coast. One year Vinny bred OG with an obscure citrus-flavored strain and called it Sunny G.[6] The breed wasn't particularly innovative, and could easily be replicated in time. But Vinny went all-in on it anyway, obtaining the naming rights to Sunny G while spending an entire summer stocking up on his new strain.

He then used his contacts in the music industry to get a few well-known local artists to name-drop Sunny G in their lyrics. When he walked into dispensaries a few months later with 200 pounds of Sunny G, Vinny was in possession of the most mysterious and sought-after strain on the market. He named his price.

The emergence of marijuana genetics, and the ease with which any talented farmer can contribute to the field, have a number of implications for the future of the industry. Most immediately, cannabis species can be bred to produce strains that suppress marijuana's psychoactive properties while drawing out its medicinal benefits.

The emergence of so many strains, each with their own unique characteristics, has also given rise to the "cannabis connoisseur"—the consumer whose knowledge of marijuana strains is both extensive and sophisticated. This development is explored in more depth in the next chapter. Suffice it to say here that an appearance of sophistication can only help to legitimize the marijuana industry as it moves closer to legalization and cultural acceptance.

But what is most interesting about the widespread proliferation of marijuana strains, in my view, is the implication it might have for the Big Marijuana prophecy that a generic takeover is inevitable. In order for a few large producers to capture the market and drive out the small-scale farmers, it wouldn't be enough to grow generic "marijuana," whatever that looks like. The Big Marijuana tycoons would need to produce massive quantities of all of the strains, on the one hand, or consumers would need to lose their appetite for choice in a market flooding them with options, on the other hand. Neither seems likely.

A common fear among small-scale farmers (and the local economies that depend on them) is that as the marijuana industry matures, the market will be flooded by generic marijuana. In other words, marijuana will become a commodity. Agricultural commodities are agricultural products that have no qualitative differentiation in the marketplace. They are fungible and treated equally with little regard for where, how, or by whom they were produced. As Karl Marx wrote, "From the taste of wheat it is not possible to tell who produced it, a Russian serf, a French peasant or an English capitalist."[7]

Commodities are not differentiated by brand, quality (or perceived quality), or sustainability of production. Besides wheat, other examples of agricultural commodities include tobacco, rye, barley, oats, cotton, soy-beans, and rice.[8] The commoditization of agricultural products allows them to be mass-produced and widely available, increasing supply and driving down prices for consumers.[9] On the other hand, by making products uniform, commoditization makes it difficult for producers and consumers to create a market for unique products.[10]

The transition from differentiated product to undifferentiated product is not black and white, as some products retain niche markets with unique characteristics, and regulations can intervene to create unique markets or prevent products from becoming commodities altogether. Eggs, for example, may be somewhere in the middle: some consumers view them as fungible and reach for the cheapest eggs available,[11] while other consumers pay more for eggs produced sustainably or ethically.[12]

States can create parallel markets by establishing regulations that impose certain requirements on otherwise fungible products. California, for example, requires all eggs sold in the state to be laid by hens raised in adequately large pens.[13] In the most aggressive cases, jurisdictions create appellations for agricultural products (such as wine or cheese), providing a protected indication based on where or how the product was created.[14]

The conventional wisdom is that, absent regulation, the marijuana industry will be dominated by large-scale, mass-produced marijuana farms that will flood the market with marijuana and drive down prices.[15] As prices drop, small-scale farming will become unprofitable, leading to consolidation of the industry into fewer farms cultivating larger quantities of marijuana.

The United States tobacco farming industry has experienced a similar process over the past several decades. While tobacco farms have traditionally been relatively small due to the labor-intensive nature of tobacco cultivation, aggregation-friendly policies and the emergence of labor-reducing technologies have led to a dramatic decline in the number of tobacco farms, in tandem with an increase in tobacco acreage per farm.[16] The trend toward fewer larger farms has made it easier for the industry as a whole to consolidate as well.[17]

Left unchecked, the marijuana industry may consolidate in similar fashion. In fact, there is evidence consolidation is taking place within states already,[18] but the truly disruptive force would be federal marijuana legalization that permits interstate marijuana commerce. As we saw in the last chapter, many states—especially California—are taking steps to prevent the farming community from being swallowed up by Big Marijuana by enacting regulations that limit the number and size of large farms. Even in an unregulated environment, however, or in states where the authorities are not interested in protecting family farms, consolidation of marijuana farms is not a given. Strains are a big reason why.

Many strains are challenging to grow and thus labor-intensive, thwarting efforts to mass-produce them. But, even if we assume large-scale agricultural methods could be adapted to a particular strain, it would be difficult to apply those methods to another strain in exactly the same way. Each strain has its own set of growing demands a farmer has to cater to. A large-scale operation could, presumably, make adjustments to cater to those demands, but small-scale farmers can make their adjustments more nimbly. That flexibility will be crucial in an industry in which consumer preferences are shifting rapidly.

As I type this, OG is one of the most dependably profitable strains on the market, and a safe investment for any farmer willing to put in the work to cultivate it. By the time you read this, however, the market may have moved on to the next latest and greatest strain, the identity of which may not be known until just before the spring planting season. Generally speaking, large agricultural operations can't make those types of wait-and-see, short-term adjustments as readily as smaller operations can.

Intellectual property law may provide small farmers and breeders with a few additional tools to defend themselves against a Big Marijuana takeover. The marijuana industry, like most others, is aggressively branded, and the branding potential within the marijuana industry may even be higher than in most other industries. Other psychoactive products, like coffee or alcohol, differentiate themselves on only two dimensions: strength and taste. But marijuana products can differentiate themselves on many dimensions, including strength, taste, method of consumption, length of consumption, and effects, to name a few. Each of these dimensions provides entrepreneurs with a branding opportunity.

Vinny's experience is a great example of the opportunities that intellectual property laws provide to farmers. Vinny's Sunny G wasn't particularly remarkable from a genetic point of view, but his branding strategy was highly effective and created strong demand for the strain. Trademark law can help small-scale farmers like Vinny prevent other farmers from calling their products "Sunny G" in hopes of capitalizing on the demand, retaining for himself the exclusive right to sell his brand.

For now, federal trademarks can't be issued for marijuana strains because marijuana remains illegal on the federal level.[19] But a trademark can be issued for the name of a marijuana strain that is used in other, legal contexts. Vinny, for example, can't trademark the name Sunny G for a marijuana strain, but he can trademark a Sunny G line of hats, shirts, or coffee mugs. In states where marijuana cultivation is legal, Vinny could also obtain a state-issued trademark for his strain of Sunny G.[20]

Patent law may be even friendlier to the marijuana industry. A patent can be issued for a new variety of plant (such as a new breed of marijuana) that provides the patent holder with exclusive rights to use, sell, or grant permission to use the plant. Plant patents come in two forms: utility patents and plant patents. Plant patents are fairly limited—they cover only the "parent plant" and its direct descendants. Utility plants cover the genetic makeup of the strain, regardless of which plants were used to create that strain. As the U.S. Patent and Trademark Office (USPTO) has explained, "to obtain a utility patent, the claimed strain must be new and unobvious over existing strains."[21]

Unlike a federal trademark, a federal patent can be issued for any number of marijuana cultivation-related inventions (including strains), despite the federal marijuana prohibition. In fact, over the past twenty-five years, around 750 cannabis-related patents have been issued. In 2015, the U.S. Patent and Trademark Office issued a patent for a psychoactive strain of marijuana for the first time, confirming that the opportunity exists for breeders and growers to patent their marijuana strains.

Granted, applying for a patent is time-consuming and potentially expensive, which might create a hurdle for small-scale entrepreneurs. But so far those hurdles haven't stopped small- to mid-size companies from becoming the most active patent applicants in the marijuana industry.[22] If Vinny can prove in his patent application that his strain of Sunny G is new and unobvious, he could obtain significant rights over the strain that, coupled with trademark protections, would provide him with a unique and branded product no one else on the market can offer to consumers.

Because small-scale farmers will continue to breed new strains of marijuana into existence, it's hard to envision a market defined by a single, generic strain of marijuana. And intellectual property law may provide these farmers with additional opportunities to ensure that their strains compete in the marketplace. They may need to lawyer up in order to realize these opportunities, but as long as marijuana remains a cash crop, it seems likely that the relative ease with which farmers can breed new strains into existence will frustrate efforts to commoditize marijuana and drive family farms out of business.

I'd like to pause here to consider three major counterarguments to this conclusion. The first is that many consumers don't care what type of strain they're consuming; they want to get high at the lowest cost possible. These consumers don't mind if their weed has a name or some fancy characteristics, but it's not the factor that matters most to them. If a generic, middle-of-the-road marijuana is available to them at the lowest price on the market, that is the marijuana they will buy.

The rise of the food movement in the United States (and its organic, eat-local, farm-to-table submovements) may give privileged cognoscenti the impression that most people want their marijuana to be unique and special and to come from a sustainable family farm, but the reality is that most consumers don't care about all that. Their most important factor when making product choices is, and will always be, price.

Jonathan Caulkins, a public policy scholar at Carnegie Mellon University and former director of the RAND Drug Policy Research Center, was quick to point out to me that his research showed most marijuana consumers in the United States have low levels of educational achievement and are mainly concerned with only two factors: price and potency. "I'm 100 percent sure there will be a niche industry to serve the rich, yuppie connoisseurs who will pay extra for hand-trimmed, organic marijuana," he told me. "But I'm acutely aware that 60 percent of consumption is by people with a high school degree or less, and what you mostly see is people going for the highest THC. ... I think the bulk of marijuana will be sold to people concerned about price."[23]

And Caulkins believes low-grade marijuana can be produced at extraordinarily low cost to the producer as well. Marijuana that "might not be suitable for sale as roll-your-own usable buds" could cost as little as $8 to $33 per pound to produce.[24] And, he estimates, if we ignored quality and environmental concerns, the entire country's marijuana demand could be supplied by a single 10,000-acre high-intensity operation.[25]

Caulkins may very well be right that a significant portion of the consumer base for marijuana cares mostly about price, and that the current landscape of production could be streamlined if the market was only concerned about achieving the lowest possible cost of production. There are a few reasons to think these facts may be accurate in general terms, but not to the extent that a Big Marijuana takeover is likely. First, while uneducated, price-driven consumers have dominated the illicit drug market in the past, today's marijuana consumers are increasingly affluent and sophisticated. A 2017 investment report on the state of the legal marijuana market observed that "the legalization, and thus legitimization, of cannabis in these markets has attracted consumers who would not, did not, or dared not participate in the illicit market previously. For the most part, these customers do not fit the mold of the traditional cannabis user. ... As these markets mature and new markets come online, expect this growing base of new or returning cannabis consumers, and their buying habits, to be more strongly felt."[26] As the consumer base changes, so too will the market's tolerance for the type of scorched-earth cultivation methods that would be necessary to achieve the lowest price possible.

Second, the production costs cited by Caulkins likely presuppose cultivation innovations that haven't emerged or been accepted by the market yet. Consider the fact that, at the moment, the going rate to have raw buds trimmed by hand is $150 to $200 per pound.[27] Machines capable of trimming those buds mechanically are available, but the quality of the trimmed buds they churn out is still so low that farmers have a hard time selling them for reasonable prices. As a result, most farmers still trim their buds by hand. Jeffrey Michael, director of the Center for Business and Policy Research at the University of the Pacific, estimates that current production costs range from $700 to $1,000 per pound.[28] Those figures are in line with the estimates I've been given by California farmers. Of course, production costs could fall with disruptive innovations or a market shift toward dirt-cheap marijuana. Until that happens, though, production costs are likely to remain stable.

Finally, even if a 10,000-acre farm capable of producing smokable marijuana with a high THC content floods the market with a generic product, most observers—like Caulkins and me—believe a high-end market for craft marijuana can thrive alongside generic products. Consumers enjoy product choice, and the thousands of marijuana strains on the market give them just that. Some may reach for the cheapest strain they can get their hands on, but the popularity of strains like OG Kush or Sour Diesel (two of the more expensive strains on the market) makes clear that the quality of the user experience remains a top priority for many consumers.

Marijuana, after all, is absorbed into your body. Unlike a product that provides a less intimate consumer experience (like paper towels, for example), it makes sense that consumers would demand marijuana that is enjoyable to smoke and isn't laden with pesticides, impurities, or synthetic fertilizers. That's especially true if the consumer base of the future isn't smoking huge quantities of marijuana every day. As Caulkins noted in our interview, "this is an industry that doesn't need to be driven by efficiency. ... The difference between corporate farming producing at ten cents per gram and small farmers producing at one dollar per gram—that may not matter to consumers very much."

Yet, when Big Marijuana believers concede that a craft market may exist for high-end marijuana, they often do so dismissively, as if a craft market is insignificant. Tim Blake, founder of the annual Emerald Cup competition that judges the best marijuana on the market, said in 2016, "these small farmers think they're going to compete against these big brands. But they're either going to have to scale up or be satisfied being the little honey stand by the side of the road."[29]

Being "the little honey stand by the side of the road" has been quite satisfactory for craft breweries situated within the commercial beer industry, which is frequently compared to the marijuana industry. In 2016, craft beer sales reached $23.5 billion, representing nearly a quarter of the country's total beer sales.[30] While the Budweisers and Coors of the industry dominate the national market, the quality and variety of beers produced by craft breweries caters to a beer-drinking public that is increasingly willing to spend a little more to drink a beer that's got some taste.

There's little reason to believe craft marijuana farmers couldn't do just as well in the marijuana industry as craft breweries do in the beer industry. Unlike microbreweries, small-scale farmers were first to capture the marijuana market—and they have a head start on the big corporations that are still waiting out the federal prohibition. Thanks to the small-scale farmers, consumers are starting to expect variety of choice and a diversity of strains to choose from. Cheap, generic marijuana will undoubtedly peel some consumers away from the high-end strains, but it would be surprising if Big Marijuana could take them all.

A related objection to my claim that marijuana genetics work in favor of small-scale farmers is that, while that may be true with respect to consumers who purchase raw buds, two of the largest sources of growth in legal markets are concentrates and edibles. Both of these product categories rely on extraction methods that pull the THC out of the marijuana plant. Concentrates often take the form of a liquid or waxy hash oil, and may have extremely high THC content (around 80 percent in some cases). The hash oil is used as is (or perhaps with some artificial flavoring) for use in vape pens and tinctures. Edibles, by contrast, incorporate hash oil into any number of food products. Common examples include gummy snacks, brownies, and spreadable butter, but there really isn't a limit to the number of foods hash oil can be added to.

Concentrates and edibles are attractive to consumers who don't enjoy inhaling smoke but still want to feel the effects of marijuana. I've met several people who shied away from a lit joint before enthusiastically accepting and eating a gummy. That mindset can be problematic—whereas the effects of inhaling marijuana smoke will hit you almost right away, edibles often take a while, tempting you to eat more. Even one edible can be more potent than anticipated, with effects that last much longer than smoking. Colorado has struggled to regulate the unanticipated rise in the marijuana edibles market, particularly among unsophisticated out-of-state tourists.[31] Regardless, the concentrates and edibles markets aren't going anywhere. In 2016, legal sales of concentrates in Colorado, Oregon, and Washington grew by 75 percent, while sales of edibles grew 53 percent.[32] As the marijuana market continues to mature, products that use hash oil are widely expected to grow in popularity and obtain a sizeable share of the product market.

The popularity of concentrates and edibles could negatively affect small-scale farmers, because when THC is being extracted and combined with food or artificial flavors, the characteristics of the marijuana it came from will feature much less than in marijuana that's consumed directly. In fact, some might say those characteristics don't feature at all. If you're eating a hash brownie designed so that the flavor of chocolate masks the flavor of marijuana, who cares what marijuana strain is in the brownie, or how the marijuana was cultivated? You might not taste the difference either way.

To put it differently, if a marijuana plant is grown for purposes of extracting its THC and producing hash oil, it may as well be grown as cheaply as possible. The fear among family farmers is that the market will forget about buds and embrace products derived from hash oil instead. Hash oil could easily be produced by a few large farms that cut every conceivable corner because no matter how unimpressive the plants turn out to be, they're all getting turned into hash oil anyway.[33] In fact, some large farms already exist solely for the purpose of producing hash oil. But the fear that hash oil will make the strain and quality of marijuana irrelevant is grossly overblown.

For one thing, hash oil often does feature the characteristics of the marijuana it was derived from. In the arms race to produce the most potent hash oil in the world, producers are creating oils with up to 90 percent THC. Admittedly, 90 percent THC oil doesn't leave much room for anything else. But if we consider the alcohol analogy again, we can see why 90 percent THC hash oil isn't necessarily a desirable product. It wouldn't be very hard to produce booze with 90 percent alcohol, but no one would drink it. The reason is simple: it would taste dreadful. By keeping alcohol levels around 40 percent, liquors like whiskey, vodka, and tequila leave some room for flavor while still packing an intoxicating punch.

The same is true for marijuana. There are at least 113 chemical compounds (called cannabinoids) in marijuana that interact with neurotransmitters in the human brain, of which THC is only one. In addition to that, marijuana contains over 100 terpenes, the biosynthetic building blocks that account for marijuana's smell and flavor. The marijuana community is only just beginning to understand the many ways in which cannabinoids and terpenes interact. It is believed that terpenes bind with THC to modify and stabilize THC absorption in your bloodstream, for example.[34] Other terpenes are responsible for working with therapeutic cannabinoids in order to relieve stress or induce sleep.

So, while it's possible to isolate THC to produce the world's most potent hash oil, there would be little reason to want to. Doing so would cause the product to lose its aroma, flavor, and, perhaps most importantly, the complex interrelationships between cannabinoids and terpenes that we barely understand. Hash oils with reasonable THC levels (say, 40 to 50 percent) will still pack a powerful punch without eliminating all the good stuff that makes marijuana so unique.

Of course, those unique characteristics are determined by the strain of the marijuana the oil was extracted from. An indica strain that has been bred to reduce anxiety will still do so in oil form. And those terpenes that give marijuana its flavor and aroma will come through in hash oil as well. So to say that making hash oil will render marijuana strains and cultivation methods irrelevant is misleading at best. Unless a consumer is purchasing a hyperconcentrated oil, the characteristics of the plant will be in the hash oil, even if they're a bit more difficult to discern. You might not taste the difference between an indica strain and a sativa strain if their oils are extracted and baked into a double chocolate brownie. But you'll darn sure *feel* the difference when the cannabinoids and terpenes start interacting with your brain.

And for all the attention concentrates and edibles are receiving due to their rise in popularity, raw buds remain the single largest product class on the market. In the legal markets of Colorado, Oregon, and Washington in 2016, raw buds accounted for 55, 57, and 59 percent of dollar sales, respectively.[35] If we add pre-rolled products to those figures,[36] they climb to 60, 64, and 69 percent of the market, respectively. Since concentrates and edibles tend to thrive in legal markets, where it's easier to market and sell packaged products, the proportion of raw buds sold on the black market is almost certain to be much higher. California's illicit marijuana trade, for example, still receives 74 percent of consumer spending on marijuana products. It would be shocking if most of that spending was on anything other than raw buds.

With legalization will come more competition from concentrates and edibles, of course. The excitement and novelty of the legal marijuana market is creating a veritable stampede to become the first to provide a niche product. While cultivating marijuana might be intimidating, marketing edibles may be less so. Countless secondary-market companies are popping up, selling everything from marijuana-flavored ice cream to marijuana-infused beard oil. As the industry matures, I expect that some of these novelties will drop out of the marketplace.

The novelties that remain will provide stiff competition to sellers of raw buds. But ultimately, producers of concentrates and edibles still need raw marijuana to make their products, and its type and quality should matter to them and their consumers. Besides, there's no reason buds, concentrates, and edibles can't coexist, because there appears to be a strong demand for all three product types. As the most foundational of the three, raw buds are well positioned to hold on to a large portion of the market. If they do, the quality and strain of those buds will retain their importance. And with that importance, the small-scale farmers growing high-grade marijuana will keep their place in the industry.

The third and final reason marijuana genetics—and the proliferation of new strains—may not be the panacea to small farmers that I think they can be is because intellectual property laws may end up working against small farmers, not for them. For one thing, patent applications are expensive, and most people don't have the expertise to file one. Lawyers may need to get involved. And obtaining a patent is only the first part of the story. In order for a patent to be useful, the patent holder has to be willing to enforce it. That means ponying up for a legal team that can identify and pursue patent infringement cases. Small-scale breeders and farmers may not have the cash or the enthusiasm to cover these ongoing legal fees.

The bigger fear, held by a small but vocal segment of the marijuana industry, is that Big Marijuana will gobble up patent rights to every strain in existence. If that happens, the best-case scenario is that every family farm in America growing marijuana would pay a license fee to grow a patented strain. In the worst-case scenario, the patent holder issues no licenses at all, reserving for itself the exclusive right to grow the country's supply of marijuana.

Utility patents are broad, and allow the patent applicant to define the scope of the claimed invention. That means a utility patent can cover the genetic makeup of the strain, as well as its traits and cultivation methods. Once issued, utility patent rights extend for twenty years, during which time other breeders would not be permitted to use that strain to breed something new. Farmers using that strain would need a license from the patent holder, and would not be permitted to use the seeds produced by the plant to grow a second generation of plants. The patented strain can't even be used in medical research without the patent holder's permission.[37]

Someone seeking a utility patent must prove that their invention is both novel (meaning it's new and hasn't been done before) and nonobvious (meaning some kind of inventive step took place).[38] Once an invention has been out in the marketplace for a year, it can no longer be patented. In theory, that should make the thousands of marijuana strains currently in existence safe from a Big Marijuana patent takeover, because none of them are new. The problem, though, is that someone has to prove it. It may be common knowledge among breeders in northern California that Trainwreck is a classic sativa-indica hybrid that farmers have been growing for years—but the U.S. Patent and Trademark Office doesn't necessarily know that. A savvy patent applicant could put together a compelling claim to have invented an existing strain and receive a patent without farmers realizing what had happened. Some might laugh at the suggestion that Trainwreck is a new invention, but they won't be laughing when they get hit with a cease and desist letter from Trainwreck's patent holder.

In a September 2017 *GQ* article, "The Great Pot Monopoly Mystery,"[39] author Amanda Chicago Lewis attempts to track down the identity and motives of a secretive company called the BioTech Institute that has been obtaining patents on marijuana strains. BioTech has quietly recruited some of the marijuana industry's foremost geneticists and is positioning itself to control marijuana agriculture by obtaining patents that would affect every marijuana strain in existence. The company has already received three utility patents, with two more patents pending. If BioTech succeeds, its patents could be worth hundreds of millions of dollars, and every marijuana farmer in America would be under its thumb. Like any good corporate mystery, the BioTech story takes Lewis down a series of dead-ends and through encounters with tight-lipped lawyers. BioTech barely exists in the public realm, and it's not clear where its money is coming from. For those in the industry keeping a watchful eye on marijuana genetics, BioTech strikes in their hearts a fear of existential proportions.

I don't doubt that legalization will bring out shadowy corporate forces, many of whom are thinking about the big picture in an effort to control the market entirely. In the battle for the heart and soul of the marijuana industry, small-scale farmers and breeders will need to take the fight to the battleground of intellectual property rights. Fortunately, some have been preparing for this battle for years.

Mowgli Holmes is one of them. His lab is one of a handful around the world that are cataloguing as many samples of marijuana as possible in an attempt to map the cannabis genome and create an archive of existing marijuana strains. The Holmes lab has already collected 2,000 specimens, and is appealing to breeders and farmers for more.[40] Holmes's goal is to put as many marijuana strains into the public domain as possible, forever protecting the marijuana community's genetic heritage from a patent takeover. When his lab's genetic database is complete, Holmes has pledged to hand it over to the Open Cannabis Project, a nonprofit organization that is putting together the world's largest open-source database of marijuana genetics. If the Open Cannabis Project can succeed in cataloguing most of the marijuana strains in existence today, it will be considerably more difficult for BioTech or any other entity to use patent law to control the market. Undoubtedly, the future of the small-scale marijuana farmer may depend on the success of grassroots efforts like this.

The breeders of the future can also obtain patents for their new strains, of course. As I've mentioned earlier, I see patent law as a powerful tool for family farmers and breeders to make their mark and stay competitive. Shell companies and corporate subsidiaries will be able to fund research and development and obtain their own patents as well, naturally. But the marijuana strains of today represent five decades of breeding and experimentation, culminating in a marketplace that is replete with thousands of genetic variations.

This foundation of genetic material—properly preserved in the public domain—has the power to provide generations of farmers with continuous access to the staggering diversity of marijuana strains their predecessors made possible. Market actors can take it from there, developing newer and better strains and obtaining patent rights if they wish. But the genetic heritage today's marijuana farmers are leaving behind may prove to be a priceless parting gift.

Many farmers I've spoken to on this topic agree with my big-picture ideas, but point out that the reality on the ground is a mess. And the central reason for this mess is inconsistency. Farmers face genetic inconsistencies in two capacities: in their attempts to reproduce plants for the next crop generation, and in their interactions with nurseries.

To understand this problem, you need to know that farmers can initiate a plant's growth in one of two ways. The most traditional method is to plant seeds. Each seed grows up to become a new plant, with a genetic makeup representing its mother and father plants. Seeded plants can grow up to become male or female, so a farmer needs to spot the difference early on and isolate the females in order to prevent them from being pollinated.

Alternatively, farmers can grow clones. A clone is a cutting taken from a mother plant, with a genetic makeup that is identical to the mother's. Any branch with a shoot, stem, and leaf can be snipped off and replanted. Clones are often taken from a single mother plant; that way, the entire crop consists of identical plants.

Which approach is better—seeds or clones—is an age-old debate. The tradeoffs are so pronounced that the farming community hasn't come close to a consensus opinion, despite decades of experience with both. Jack is a good example, a living microcosm of the industry's tension on the subject.

In 2017, Jack's marijuana crops consisted entirely of clones. Yet, as he told me, "seeds are better, hands down."

Indeed, the case for seeds is compelling. Seeded plants, in general, are more vigorous than clones. They grow faster and stronger, so their stems and branches aren't as likely to break. Seeded plants grow bigger and yield more buds. Their root system is stronger and deeper, and require water less often. Compared to clones, which often carry pests and the diseases of their mothers with them, seeded plants are a clean slate. A seed can be planted in the ground much earlier in the spring planting season, since it won't be confused by spring's shorter photoperiods as a more biologically mature clone would.[41] Seeded plants are, overall, easier to grow, due to a process called senescence. The journal *Nature* defines senescence as "the process by which cells irreversibly stop dividing and enter a state of permanent growth arrest."[42] To put it more simply, the biological integrity of complex lifeforms deteriorates over time. Plants are no different, becoming less vigorous with age. Both seeded plants and clones experience senescence (like all plants); the difference is that clones are much further along in the aging process than seeds. A seed represents a completely new lifeform. When it is planted, it is at the first stage of its life cycle, and grows into the world with the vitality of youth.

Clones are a bit different. Cut from an established female plant, clones are already biologically mature. A clone will continue to grow when cut and reestablished on its own, but it won't grow with the same vigor as a plant grown from seed. To make matters worse, many clones are taken from a single mother plant that is used year after year. Or a clone will be taken from a mother plant that is herself a clone too.

Imagine that a farmer grows a big beautiful female plant from seed, and decides to take some cuttings from her to establish identical clones for the next growing season. Then, of those clones, the farmer chooses one to make the next batch of clones (it doesn't matter which one since they're all genetically identical). Each year thereafter the farmer takes cuttings from one of the previous year's clones. If the farmer repeats this process for ten years, the newest batch of clones, despite looking like young plants, would have experienced the senescence of a ten-year-old plant.[43] They will be small, weak, and low-yielding.

For this reason, clones can never be too many generations removed from a seeded plant, otherwise the senescence becomes too extreme. So there should always be a market for seeds.[44] The question is, if seeded plants are so much more vigorous compared to clones—if they really are "better, hands down," as Jack claims—why bother with clones in the first place? Why not start plants from seed every time? Why is Jack growing a crop composed entirely of clones?

The answer: consistency. Seeds are the product of two plants reproducing and creating something new. A farmer can't know what a seed will grow up to be until it has grown up to be it. As a preliminary matter, around half the plants will grow up to become males that consumed valuable resources and nonetheless need to be removed.[45] Clones taken from a female, by contrast, will grow up to be female.[46] The seeded females that are left will still be, by nature, genetically different from one another, even if they share the same parents. Ideally those differences are minute, but often the differences are significant enough that when the crop is harvested, it consists of a collection of buds that can't be sold as the same product.

Consider a farmer whose goal is to grow 100 plants of Sour Diesel. He'd start by pollinating a vigorous Sour Diesel female with the pollen of a Sour Diesel male. In order to ensure a 100-plant crop, the farmer would need to plant a little over 200 seeds. Half the crop will consist of males the farmer eliminates, leaving him with 100 Sour Diesel females, the original goal. But, of those 100, perhaps only eighty produce buds that a dispensary or wholesale buyer would unmistakably recognize as high-grade Sour Diesel. The rest are more or less Sour Diesel, but in today's hypercompetitive marketplace, more or less doesn't cut it. It's either Sour Diesel as the market has come to expect it, or it isn't.

The farmer can still sell the "more or less" buds, but not at the same price as the purer buds. The farmer could also keep the "more or less" buds and turn them into hash oil. Though the farmer has options, consistency is king. Even if the seeded crop yields buds that are similar in quality, the crop will be hard to sell if the buds look different. Buyers want a consistent product, and seeded plants can't guarantee that.

Clones are all about consistency, since they are exact genetic replicas. If the farmer in the example above had instead taken 100 cuttings from the vigorous Sour Diesel female, his plants would have matured into a crop of identical Sour Diesel females. They might have been smaller, weaker, and less vigorous than the seeded plants, and the farmer might have needed to spend more time caring for them, watering them, or ridding them of pests. They might have yielded fewer buds. But when the farmer harvested their buds, the yield of the whole crop could be packaged together and sold as the same product, because the buds would all look the same. They would all look like Sour Diesel.

Other industries have realized the potential of cloning. Winemakers often use clones when laying out their vineyards. If they didn't, a vineyard of 100 vines would produce a wine with 100 different flavor profiles. Jack's Syrah vines, for example, are all clones of the same mother vine. That way his wine stays balanced and consistent. Lavender is cultivated with clones for similar reasons: when consumers smell a bundle of lavender, they want to smell one terrific lavender smell, not a bevy of aromas in conflict with each other.

Ultimately, it's up to each farmer to determine which method works best for him or her. There isn't an easy answer. And to make matters more difficult, farmers also need to determine where to obtain the seeds or clones they want to use. Sometimes a farmer can take care of her own needs if she already has a vigorous female she wants to clone or pollinate. But the speed with which the market creates demand for new strains forces even the most insular grower to leave the farm on occasion. And that's where nurseries come in.

Marijuana nurseries act as a hub for the growing community. They get farmers started at the beginning of the growing season by selling seeds, seeded starts, or clones. They act as bellwethers, keeping tabs on strains in demand and adjusting their stock accordingly. And they can also be gatekeepers, influencing which strains will be available in a given year. Nurseries take many different forms. A few have distinguished themselves as large, reputable operations, selling thousands of clones and starts every year. Other nurseries operate on a smaller, more regional or local scale. Dispensaries often maintain a nursery as part of their business. Some businesses are exclusively seed distributors. And in many cases, "nursery" is a loose term for a friend who took more clones off a mother plant than she needed and is willing to share.

The problem that all of these nursery businesses have in common is consistency. For the time being, there's no way to identify the strain when you're looking at a seed. Ditto for a clone or seed start. When marijuana plants are young, they all look pretty much the same. At some point the Open Cannabis Project or something similar might be able to provide a genetic certification process, but until then farmers have no choice but to take a chance with the nursery they buy from. Every farmer I've talked to has been burned on occasion. One farmer bought fifty clones of Durban Poison from a nursery, but a few weeks later it became clear that only thirty of those plants were truly Durban Poison. Another farmer bought a large batch of Grape Ape clones that grew into plants so weak they couldn't support themselves.

There are also risks inherent in keeping thousands of clones together in the same space. One large and otherwise reputable nursery in northern California is known to have russet mites, a pest that can devastate a marijuana crop. A clone cut from a mother plant that has russet mites will likely have russet mites itself, but an infestation can be hard to see when you're buying a few hundred small plants. When a friend of Jack's called the nursery to complain about the mites, the nursery allegedly responded that their methods are organic and mites should be expected. Another nursery has an online menu of strains that doesn't match their actual inventory. When a farmer put himself on the waiting list for a one-month-back-ordered strain, he didn't get a call from the nursery until three months later, well past the planting season.

Some of these problems might be expected of an industry that is new and finding its way through the murky legalization process. Not everyone becomes a professional entrepreneur overnight, after all. But if the government doesn't step in to regulate nurseries or a third-party certifier doesn't emerge organically, the farming community will continue to be held back by inconsistencies in the seed and clone supply chain. Unfortunately, with the rise of social media, that problem appears to be getting worse, not better.

Now that breeders, nurseries, and dispensaries have less fear of prosecution than ever before, many are taking advantage by developing large and profitable social media profiles. For example, a breeder will post a picture of a beautiful bud of a brand-new strain on his Instagram account. The picture is accompanied by a flowery description of the strain's characteristics, and where a farmer can buy the seeds. The more common this practice becomes, the more pressure these businesses feel to keep offering new strains. That in itself is not a bad thing, for the reasons I've discussed throughout this chapter. But in the rush to develop the latest and greatest new strains, breeders are forgetting about backcrossing.

The first time a new strain is created, its direct lineage will be unstable. Pollinate Northern Lights (an indica) with Green Crack (a sativa), and the seeds that come out will produce plants that are all over the map. Some may resemble the Northern Lights, others the Green Crack. One of those plants might produce the hybrid a breeder is looking for, and that plant can be cloned to reproduce those buds for a few generations. But in order to propagate the strain indefinitely (and establish the strain on the market), the breeder needs the plant to produce seeds. The breeder could take one of the hybrid males and breed it with the hybrid female, but the descendants of that pair may not come out like the female, and likely won't.

Backcrossing is the process of breeding a hybrid with one of its parents in order to create descendants that reliably feature the characteristics of the parent. In this case, instead of breeding the hybrid female with a hybrid male, the breeder can breed the hybrid female with the original Northern Lights male. One of the males produced by that pair can then breed with the original Green Crack female. Repeat this process over and over, each time backcrossing with one of the original parents, and eventually the strain stabilizes into a hybrid that reliably features the characteristics the breeder is looking for.

The downside of backcrossing is that it takes time. In their rush to put new strains on the market, many breeders aren't willing to spend a year or two backcrossing in order to stabilize the genetics of the strain. By the time farmers find out the strain is unstable and can't produce consistent buds, the transaction has already taken place. Back in the day, reputation and word of mouth would take care of this issue, but the influx of new entrants to the market that comes along with legalization is obscuring a number of inefficiencies. The inconsistent products put out by nurseries and breeders is one of them.

Jack, like any good entrepreneur, sees this inefficiency as a business opportunity. When he applied for a cultivation license from the state in 2016, the application form required him to indicate which business activities he wanted a license for. Though Jack hadn't given it much thought before, when he saw the box for "nursery," he thought, "why not?" He'd had good relationships with local nurseries in the past, but the green rush was straining their capabilities, and loyal customers were increasingly dealing with stock shortages and inconsistent seeds, starts, and clones. Jack had already decided that he would, for the most part, take matters into his own hands in 2017 and beyond. And if he was prepared to invest in his own nursery, it seemed a good idea to leave himself the option to sell to others as well.

With profit margins getting smaller and smaller, Jack didn't have much excess cash on hand at the end of the 2017 harvest. His plants had produced to his expectations, and buyers were impressed with his product. But the price per pound had dropped precipitously from the previous year, while Jack's costs had remained the same. But Jack has never been one to sit still, especially not while the market moved forward. So he made a bold move, investing most of his remaining capital into a 4,000-square-foot multipurpose facility, what he calls "the barn."

One side of the barn houses his winemaking equipment, including a press, crusher, and bottler. On the other side sits the nursery. The nursery holds row upon row of lighted shelving, growing hundreds of clones. The facility is large enough that Jack could cultivate as many clones and seed starts as the local growing community can demand. And now, crucially, Jack's business can operate year-round, no longer limited by northern California's cold, wet winters.

The barn isn't the only risk Jack took on that winter. He, too, struggles with the "seeds or clones" conundrum. And now that he's running a nursery business, his reputation is on the line to produce the consistency growers are looking for. He needed to think outside the box.

Though he dropped out of college to pursue a career in the marijuana industry, Jack has always been gifted when it comes to math and science. He impressed his college geology teacher so much in the classroom that she invited him to an exclusive meet-and-greet with the oil and gas industry's top scientists. Jack arrived at the event in dreadlocks, a hoodie, and the insouciance of youth that, collectively, made him irresistibly intriguing. He was offered a job on the spot—$120,000 a year for three years, plus a $20,000 signing bonus. All he had to do was graduate. He turned it down without so much as a consultation with his friends and family. When he casually mentioned the job offer to me a few months later, the most I could get out of him was, "I don't know. Just wasn't interested."

Botany, on the other hand, commands Jack's full attention. The science of growing plants fascinates him to the point that he'll spend hours chatting with a vintner in Napa County, picking her brain for tips that can help him grow better grapes and make better wine. You get the impression he believes there's a solution to every roadblock that plants can put in his way. So when it came to this "seeds or clones" roadblock, he's been on the alert for a breakthrough. And he may have found it with a technique that was first proposed in 1902 by an Austrian botanist named Gottlieb Haberlandt.

In the late nineteenth century, Gottlieb Haberlandt was a well-recognized expert in plant physiology, with a particular interest in the reproduction of plant cells.[47] In 1902, he was invited to deliver an address to the German

Academy of Science. During the address, Haberlandt discussed his recent experiments isolating plant cells, many of which were interesting but unsuccessful in their attempts to foster growth. But Haberlandt's philosophical mind could see the implications of his work despite the failure of his experiments. He proposed to the Academy that, in theory, "all plant cells are able to give rise to a complete plant."[48] From this proposal emerged the concept of totipotency. A single cell, Haberlandt believed, could be taken from a plant and cultivated into a new plant. Though Haberlandt was never able to substantiate his theory, the next generation of botanists proved he was right. The propagation of clones via cell cultivation—now referred to as plant tissue culture—is a commonly used technique in a wide variety of applications, including commercial floriculture, forestry, and endangered species conservation. If you can isolate cells in a sterile medium (such as a petri dish), they will, eventually, grow up to become a full-grown mature plant.

Talk to marijuana farmers about tissue culture, and many of them will give you a blank stare—but that may be about to change. At least two nurseries in northern California have attempted to cultivate clones by tissue culturing. One nursery couldn't pull it off, but the other is enjoying impressive results. And now Jack plans on building a laboratory capable of hosting a commercial tissue culture operation. If he succeeds, the "seeds or clones" debate may become obsolete.

As we know, a clone cut from a mother plant gives farmers the crop consistency they need to sell a uniform product, but the tradeoff is that clones tend to lack vigor and resilience. A crop of seeded plants will be vigorous and resilient, but the product won't be uniform. Tissue culture may represent the best of both worlds. When a cell is taken from a mother plant and cultured in a medium, it replicates the genetic makeup of its mother, thereby making it a clone. But, whereas a cutting is biologically mature and vulnerable to senescence, pests, and diseases, a tissue-cultured plant represents a clean slate. It grows with the vigor of a seeded plant, cleared of its mother's pests and diseases. And while a mother plant can only provide so many cuttings, a steady hand with a scalpel could remove a nearly limitless supply of cell tissues. After all, as Haberlandt predicted, all you need is a single cell.

The science of tissue culturing is remarkable, and a testament to the reproductive powers of the plant kingdom. And yet the practice is well established and commercially successful in other contexts. Its application to marijuana agriculture is not yet fully understood, but there doesn't appear to be any reason it couldn't end the "seeds or clones" debate once and for all. True, the technique requires precision and a sterile laboratory, which isn't a common feature of the average marijuana farm. But for people like Jack who are willing to embrace it, tissue culture may represent an opportunity to provide the farming community with, as he puts it, "clones that aren't shitty."

For the small-scale farming community to reach its potential, it will need to iron out the inefficiencies that might prevent it from competing with the well-funded corporate agribusinesses. The inconsistencies provided by seeded plants, on the one hand, and nurseries, on the other hand, are two such inefficiencies. Time will tell if tissue culture allows the farming community to overcome these issues.

The more I learn about cannabis species, the more convinced I am that marijuana is not destined to become the commodity so many predict it will become. Marijuana plants are capable of so much diversity that it starts to feel silly to use the word "marijuana" as a catchall term in the first place. The plant's potential genetic diversity has allowed marijuana breeders to create thousands of strains, each with a unique set of characteristics and effects on the consumer. This genetic diversity will make it difficult to commoditize marijuana, and should, at the very least, leave room for a craft farming community to provide a variety of high-end, artisanal strains to consumers.

A plant's genetic makeup, however, represents only its potential. A farmer still needs to realize that potential by cultivating it to maturity. Along the way, a number of factors—including the soil, climate, photoperiod, and agricultural support—influence the characteristics of the final product. Grape growers and winemakers have built a lucrative wine industry by harnessing this fact and using it to their advantage. Can marijuana farmers do the same?

6 The Marijuana Appellation

No nation is drunken where wine is cheap; and none sober, where the dearness of wine substitutes ardent spirits as the common beverage.

—Thomas Jefferson, third president of the United States[1]

Cabot's Cab is probably very much of its place, along the Klamath River in Humboldt County: quite savory, with flavors of leather, tobacco and cranberry around a middleweight texture and tight tannins.

—*Wine Enthusiast* review of Cabot Vineyards 2007 Cabernet Sauvignon[2]

Bubba Kush is an indica strain that has gained notoriety in the U.S. and beyond. …Sweet hashish flavors with subtle notes of chocolate and coffee come through on the exhale, delighting the palate.…Bubba Kush exhibits a distinctive, bulky bud structure with hues that range from forest green to pale purple.…Bubba Kush emerged just after 1996,…[and] has flourished from its California roots ever since.

—Leafly.com review of marijuana strain Bubba Kush[3]

1890 was a bad year for Champagne. A sap-sucking insect called phylloxera had already wiped out scores of French vineyards during a period that came to be known as the Great French Wine Blight. And now the pest was making its presence known in Champagne's prized winemaking industry, just when the region was riding high. The Belle Époque had ushered in an era of economic prosperity in France, and champagnes—well established as luxury goods favored by nobles such as King Louis XIV and Napoleon Bonaparte—were in demand. Phylloxera weakened Champagne, preventing the region from meeting the rise in demand.

To make matters worse, inferior regions and fraudulent winemakers were taking advantage of Champagne's hard-earned reputation—and moment of weakness—by selling counterfeit champagne. Just three years earlier, Champagne's top producers had banded together to combat the fraudsters, winning a court battle against winemakers in the Loire Valley who were marketing their sparkling wines as champagne.[4] But fake champagne was streaming in from all directions. Even winemakers in Champagne were taking advantage, importing cheap grapes from other regions under cover of their local wine label.

Tensions carried over into the twentieth century, when prolific counterfeiting combined with several poor harvests in Champagne. Relations between wine regions were becoming volatile, potentially explosive. The French government had to act before the country turned on itself. Its solution was to enact geographic designation rules, preventing anyone outside of a region from using the region's name on their products. Riots broke out almost immediately, with winemakers all over the country upset about the boundaries being drawn, and the implications they would have for their labels. It was an agricultural class war, pitting regions against one another.

Finally in 1911 the boundaries were drawn to accommodate more territory into the designated region of Champagne, and tensions eased as World War I redefined the enemy for a while. But in the interwar years, Champagne producers were at war once again, and this time with themselves. While the protected designations of origin system prevented outsiders from using the Champagne name on their wines, nothing prevented Champagne producers from exploiting the region's sterling reputation by making poor-quality champagne and pocketing the extra profits. With each winemaker facing a similar incentive, the region was at risk of losing its pristine status atop the world of wine.

The government responded by creating the Institut National des Appellations d'Origine (INAO), an agency tasked with creating and enforcing cultivation and production guidelines for Champagne and every other region in France. The INAO ensured that each region's rules maintained a certain standard of quality. And at the same time, the INAO stood watch on behalf of its regions, making sure that a region's name was used only by the region's own producers.

The benefits of the system were numerous. Regions enjoyed a measure of economic protection from foreign imposters. The marketplace offered a diversity of unique products. Wine quality improved. Product labels became more reliable and informative for consumers. A niche connoisseur market emerged. Not everyone enjoyed the benefits of a Champagne designation, but the battle to protect its name created a rare win-win for winemakers all over France.

The idea caught on quickly all over Europe.[5] It is now the dominant organizational model of the European Union, with protections covering dozens of agricultural products. Eventually the rest of the world embraced the system as well, incorporating the model into the World Trade Organization's global trade regime. The seductive appeal of protecting designations of origin could not be denied. The appellation had arrived.

Strictly speaking, an appellation is a legally protected geographical indication used to identify where an agricultural product comes from.[6] To use the name of an appellation on a product, a producer must meet the appellation's geographic or quality standards.[7] If a winemaker wants to put "Napa Valley" on her wine label, for example, a certain percentage of the grapes used to make the wine must have been grown in Napa Valley, California. Some type of regulatory body is responsible for setting the rules and making sure they are met: in one jurisdiction, appellations may be regulated by a national government agency; in others, appellations are self-governed. In the latter case, the producers in the region get together to set the standards and ensure compliance.

Appellations are most commonly associated with the wine industry, but they can be applied to any agricultural product for which the geographic origin carries importance. The wine industry's success with appellations is due, in part, to the assumption that environmental conditions influence the quality and character of a grape (and it is generally agreed that this assumption has merit).[8] The finished wine, therefore, exhibits qualities that are unique to the region that produced the grapes contained in the wine. These environmental conditions—for example, the soil, aridity, and temperature of the vineyard—are collectively referred to as the *terroir*. Because the terroir of a wine comes through when you drink it, it makes sense to regulate the industry along geographic lines. But a terroir isn't necessary in order to protect designations of origin; it is enough that a region makes a quality product and wants to restrict outsiders from associating their products with the region's reputation.

An appellation's product standards always have geographic requirements, and some have quality or production requirements as well. Quality standards tend to increase the quality of grapes grown in the appellation, improving wine quality and the region's reputation.[9] Production standards may require that a certain method be used during production, which could be designed to maintain tradition or quality (by preventing anyone from cutting corners).

Generally speaking, appellations in the United States do not have stringent cultivation rules, and speak more to the geographic origin of the product than to the product's quality. American wine appellations, composed of states, counties, or American Viticultural Areas (AVAs), are regulated by the Treasury Department's Alcohol and Tobacco Tax and Trade Bureau (TTB).[10] The AVA model requires only that wines using an appellation designation actually come from that appellation region.[11]

In contrast to American appellation designations which indicate geographic origin only, the French appellation model, like some others, allows the appellation designation only if stringent cultivation rules and regulations are followed, ensuring that wines carrying appellation designations meet high quality standards.[12] There are tradeoffs characteristic to both systems. The French model provides quality assurance at the cost of agricultural freedom, whereas the U.S. model fosters innovation but fails to convey any nongeographic information.

In either case, as the reputation of a region's agricultural product grows, the appellation designation creates a unique market for the product, increasing prices while precluding other producers from associating their products with the region.[13] Appellations therefore create mandatory differentiation in the market, frustrating efforts to commoditize the industry. This can be beneficial to local economies that are threatened by cheap alternatives to their products.[14] The European Union's appellations law explicitly declares that benefit to be a primary objective of its designation of origin protections.[15] Appellations promote the development of unique and high-quality products in the marketplace by providing farmers and producers with a fair price for their efforts,[16] which in turn provides a boost to rural economies and keeps rural populations stable. For the European Union, appellations are a key to agricultural and rural development.

Protectionism of local industries and their brands has a secondary benefit: by certifying that products with geographic indicators are accurately designated, appellations assure consumers of authenticity. When Champagne experienced crop failures in 1890, fraudulent producers from other regions attempted to replace the resulting drop in supply by selling lower-quality wine and passing it off as champagne.[17] This harmed real champagne producers, of course, but consumers suffered as well—they were paying inflated prices for a low-quality product. Today, AVAs assure consumers of American wine that the wine they are purchasing actually originates where it claims to. In other appellation systems with more rigorous cultivation requirements, the designations can communicate information about the product's quality, rarity, or sustainability standards.[18]

These twin goals of providing economic benefits (by promoting rural development) and consumer protection (by conveying information and authenticity) underlie the basic motivations of most appellation systems.[19] There are drawbacks to appellation systems, naturally. Most obvious are the administrative costs of imposing a regulatory system on agricultural products that could be cultivated, marketed, sold, and consumed without any reference to the place of origin. The French appellation system, for instance, is notoriously bureaucratic, requiring producers to collectively develop and enforce a unique set of cultivation standards.[20] Despite these costs, however, the thoughtful, bottom-up development of cultivation standards offers tangible benefits in itself. The process of creating and maintaining appellations brings agricultural producers together to negotiate or address regional issues, and there is evidence that appellations promote more sustainable and ecologically responsive practices.[21]

Products protected by a designation of origin can coexist with cheaper generics and agricultural commodities, of course, as consumers demand goods in a variety of formats and permutations. The problem is that intellectual property laws don't protect a region's name or products from being counterfeited by outsiders. Without protection, it becomes impossible for a region to capitalize on its reputation. Without protection, farmers and producers aren't fairly compensated for creating unique, high-quality products. And without protection, consumers can't be sure of the authenticity of product labels.

Fortunately, geographic protections are in place for many agricultural products. Appellation systems are well established all over the world, and in most cases appear to be working exceedingly well. Farmers and producers are receiving higher returns for their geographically designated products, in part because consumers are willing to pay more for products that are reliably unique.[22] It is a win-win-win for farmers, consumers, and market diversity.

Allow me to illustrate the power of appellations with a personal anecdote. The setting: Christmas Eve day, 2016, Aix-en-Provence, France. The French side of my family—my mother's side—is gathered together in the living room of an apartment we've rented for the holidays. It's a crisp, sunny, late afternoon in the south of France, and the empty bottles of champagne accumulating in the kitchen present a rather incriminating case that we're having a particularly good time. Luxury goods aren't a common presence in this family, but on special occasions we, like many families all over France, splurge on good food and good wine. A few days earlier, my uncle François came down from Grenoble with a whole case of champagne, delighting the rest of us with anticipation.

But, as the late afternoon sun starts to set on Christmas Eve, my brother begins to open the last bottle left in the case. My father stops him, proposing we save the bottle for later, seemingly under the impression that we've had enough.[23] This does not go over well with the crowd. But the logic of having some champagne on hand for an as-yet-unascertained future date is undeniably compelling. Solidly in the "open it" camp, I suggest a third option to resolve the dilemma: why not go to the wine store and buy some reinforcements? Before the matter can be put up for debate, I'm flying out the door, skipping steps on my way down to the street.

A few moments later, standing in front of a wall of champagnes, I realize what many a novice wine enthusiast has realized before me. Champagne ain't cheap, even in France. I ask the gentleman behind the register for some guidance, explaining that in an ideal world I'd leave the store with some change left in my pocket. He points out a few mid-priced champagnes, then steers me to an adjacent wall. "*Crémant de Bourgogne*," he says. Sparkling wine produced in Burgundy, a well-respected wine region along Champagne's southern border.

Crémants are made using the *méthode champenoise*, the traditional champagne production method that requires a secondary fermentation in the bottle. Many of them also use the same grape varietals that champagne-makers use, just that they're grown a few miles to the south. Crémants aren't cheap (they're now the second most expensive sparkling wines in France, after champagne), in part because the appellation imposes strict cultivation and winemaking protocols to keep quality high. But a crémant doesn't carry the same luxury tax a champagne bottle does, the gentleman explained. "Sounds good to me," I thought. I grabbed a crémant and one of the mid-priced champagnes off the shelf. *"Parfait,"* said the gentleman. *"Joyeux Noël."*

I hurried back to the apartment just in time to keep the momentum of the festivities going. Both bottles were put on ice, and the champagne was opened and enjoyed in short order. When my uncle pulled out the crémant, a subtle look of confusion came over his face. *Not a champagne,* I could tell he was thinking (this is the moment I start doubting my purchase). Ever tactful, he opened the bottle anyway and refilled our glasses. But when my grandfather leaned in for his share, my uncle made sure he knew what he was getting. *"Ah. Non alors,"* my grandfather said as he pulled back his glass. *"Je mélange pas le champagne."* Thanks, but no thanks, he was saying. "I don't mix champagne." And that was the moment I start regretting my purchase.

Of all the mistakes I've made in my life, my error in purchasing a crémant doesn't top the list, I'll readily admit. But I was disappointed in myself. The rest of my family drank the crémant respectfully, but my grandfather—a man I've idolized since I was a child—was steadfast in his refusal. The matter-of-fact tone with which he explained himself made clear his position wasn't personal, he just doesn't mix alcohol, is all. And to be fair, while a Crémant de Bourgogne might employ the *méthode champenoise*, and use similar grapes grown in a similar region, it's a well-known fact that crémants and champagnes can taste very different. One crémant winemaker described the two wines as "cabbage and carrots—the same class of wine, but completely different from one another."[24]

Can I taste the difference? Maybe a little, but that wouldn't stop me from drinking a good crémant. "Tastes great to me," my father agreed reassuringly. But my grandfather is ninety-four years old, with a discerning taste that was cultivated in his native France. If anyone can tell the difference between the two wine regions, it's him. And after a lifetime of drinking good wines, he'd rather not drink at all than confuse his palate.

I paid a price for saving money—which is exactly what an effective appellation system is designed to do. Bring a bottle of champagne to a party, and you'll get a reaction no other wine can elicit. Appellations can be used for quality control, but they're just as capable of providing brand control and name recognition. This is as true for wine as it is for other products, like cheese, olive oil, or cured meat. The protected designation of origin differentiates the product and creates exclusivity. Mandatory quality controls or a region's reputation do the rest.

There's no reason this arrangement couldn't work for the marijuana industry. Consumers could embrace commoditization and consolidation of cultivation, of course, providing everyone with cheap and plentiful marijuana.[25] The industry could, alternatively, reject that approach in favor of a marijuana appellation system that encourages the development of diverse farming regions and high-quality products. The cheap generic stuff will continue to exist (Big Marijuana will make sure of that). But consumers will also have regionally protected marijuana products to choose from, as well as the security of knowledge that the products' designations of origin are authentic.

The current state of American marijuana farming exhibits many of the characteristics that make an agricultural product a natural fit for appellations. First, while a terroir isn't necessary to justify protecting a designation of origin, whenever a region's environment really does make a difference in the final product, a geographic marker is a logical means of capitalizing on that. While it isn't clear if marijuana has a terroir, early indications suggest that it might. A research team at Portland State University has been testing marijuana plants to find evidence of terroir. Their preliminary results have exciting implications for marijuana agriculture:

> While the genotype determines the range of possible traits that a plant may have, growth conditions determine where they will be on the spectrum of possibilities. … The presence of specific organic compounds seems tied to genetics, [but] preliminary data suggest that the relative abundance of those compounds among plants from unique farms may be related to differences in growing methods and terroir.[26]

The terroir of marijuana, if strong enough for discerning consumers to detect, may give rise to a robust connoisseur market. That market already exists with respect to marijuana strains, but terroir may create an additional layer of sophistication for high-end consumers.

Even if marijuana's terroir is negligible, the environmental conditions of a region dictate which marijuana strains are suitable for cultivation. Indica strains thrive in northern California because the arid climate allows indicas to produce their characteristically large, dense buds without attracting mold or mildew. In Jamaica, by contrast, marijuana farmers cultivate sativa strains that are accustomed to tropical humidity and temperatures.[27] Seed companies have responded to these realities by marketing strains to match a diversity of outdoor conditions.[28]

Instead of competing with one another to produce the most popular generic strains, appellations allow regions to embrace the strains that grow well in their environment. France's Burgundy and Northern Rhône regions are well known for growing pinot noir and Syrah grape varietals, respectively.[29] Neither region is threatened by outside producers or forced to adopt ill-suited varietals because they have created individual markets for their own well-respected grapes. The same could be true of marijuana farming regions.

A second reason appellations are a promising model for the marijuana industry is that regional marijuana farming cultures are developing across the country due to the persistent federal marijuana prohibition. While the U.S. government's enforcement of its own marijuana laws may be inconsistent, the federal prohibition is effectively preventing legal marijuana markets from engaging in interstate commerce. Black-market trade is still prolific, and crosses state lines. But legal supply chains are strong enough that whenever a state legalizes marijuana use, an in-state agricultural sector must emerge to supply consumers with the legal marijuana that only in-state farmers can provide. And state governments, of course, have a strong incentive to protect their regional farming industries.

In the case of other agricultural products, the product may be grown wherever a region has captured the market first or wherever a crop grows most efficiently. But in the case of marijuana, until the federal prohibition is lifted, plants must be grown in states with a legal market and cannot be sold across state lines. If the trend continues uninterrupted, each state in America will have a constituency of legal marijuana farmers.

When the federal prohibition is eventually lifted and Big Marijuana threatens to flood the national market with cheap, generic marijuana, will states sit idly by while their constituents are driven out of business? Or will they take steps to protect their farmers and rural economies? If states choose the latter, appellations would be an effective tool. Appellations won't be needed to create a national landscape of marijuana farming regions; they'll just be needed to protect the landscape that already exists.

As regional reputations develop, appellations will be needed to protect those reputations from fraudulent appropriation. After all, reputations can be monetized. This somewhat obvious fact is what makes appellations appealing to a region with a strong reputation. Individual brand names can be protected through trademark protections and intellectual property rights, but appellations are needed to protect and monetize the name[30] of an entire region or group of producers.

The reputation of the Champagne region in France would be worth much less to champagne producers there if anyone anywhere can slap the word "champagne" on their product. Not only would the "champagne" label become less rare and therefore less valuable (since anyone could use it), but the region's reputation would suffer as low-quality products attached themselves to its name. By restricting use of the name "champagne" to the Champagne region's producers, Champagne products remain exclusive (and therefore expensive) and the region retains control over the quality of its product, and therefore its reputation.

You don't need to look very far to find examples of regional reputation in the marijuana industry. Look at references in the music industry, to use just one example. The reputation of marijuana-producing regions is repeatedly mentioned (and reinforced) in the lyrics of some of the world's biggest music stars. Toby Keith, the country music star whose discography includes twelve platinum albums, wrote in his song "Wacky Tobaccy": "You got your Mexican and Jamaican with those buds of blue / Humboldt County and hydroponic too / Okeechobee purple from down in the south."[31] In three lines, Keith manages to name-drop three marijuana-producing regions (Mexico, Jamaica, and Humboldt County) and one strain (Okeechobee Purple). Rock band 311 made a similar reference to Humboldt County in their song "Nutsymptom": "I puff on the stuff of a Humboldt cone / Then I'm stoned, watch out / Smoke the weed that come from Northern California."[32] Grammy award-winning R&B star Ashanti likens Humboldt County marijuana to love itself: "Now if I was trying to hold in this love, I would choke / Cause it's some potent shit like from Humboldt County on the West Coast."[33] The phrase "Cali weed" has become synonymous with quality marijuana, thanks to repeated references in hip hop lyrics. Redman, rap star and platinum-album producer himself, drops the following lines in his song "Blow Treez": "Smokin' on that Sour Dies' / That cali weed's / So funky we call it cottage cheese."[34]

Other examples include songs by Nas ("so I keep the Cali weed in the bong and I'm strong"),[35] Wiz Khalifa ("that's that Cali weed, I know that smell anywhere";[36] "Cali weed blowing like a Rastaman, Kush seed straight from Afghanistan"[37]), and Master P ("Cali got that good ass weed, that good ass weed, that good ass weed").[38] Dr. Dre, Snoop Dogg, Wu-Tang Clan, Lil Wayne, Rick Ross, 50 Cent, R. Kelly, and Jay-Z have made similar references in their songs as well.

The list of popular culture citations goes on, of course, including references in books, movies, and TV. All of it is free advertising and endorsement of the highest order. Plus, each time a region is mentioned—be it Humboldt County, northern California, or the entire state of California—the region's brand and reputation are reinforced.

All of this is great, but it doesn't translate into a material benefit for the region if a novice basement grower in Arkansas can claim that his low-grade marijuana comes from Humboldt County, too. The Arkansas grower would be benefiting from the reputation built by Humboldt farmers, while simultaneously diluting the brand and associating the region with an inferior product. It's the same trick fraudsters used in nineteenth-century France to impersonate Champagne. And make no mistake, whether you're impersonating Humboldt marijuana or Champagne sparkling wine, the trick works—unless the region fights to protect itself.

Analysts can see that brand is "a huge factor in consumer purchasing decisions" within legal marijuana markets.[39] Pop culture references to "cali weed" suggest that the geographic origin of marijuana has been a large factor in consumer purchasing decisions on the black market for some time now, as well. When federal legalization allows interstate commerce for marijuana products, regions will need a mechanism to protect their brand. Certifying a designation of origin by adopting an appellation system represents a mechanism that is designed to do exactly that.

Finally, the information that appellations communicate to consumers would be a welcome feature for the marijuana industry. Because marijuana has been (and in many jurisdictions continues to be) cultivated and sold on the black market, consumers have traditionally had little to no information on where or how their marijuana was grown. That this lack of information can be problematic for unsuspecting consumers is illustrated by the paraquat-contaminated marijuana coming from Mexico in the 1970s. No one would be stupid enough to consume paraquat willingly, a fact the cartels dealt with by concealing the true nature of their product.

Marijuana continues to enter the market from dubious sources, including Mexico.[40] Given the well-publicized violence and corruption associated with Mexican drug cartels,[41] it is not unreasonable to believe consumer behavior would reflect a preference for domestically grown marijuana if geographic designations were reliable. In fact, there is evidence that legal marijuana cultivation in the United States is already driving "cartel grows" out of business.[42] Since marijuana has illicit dimensions in many jurisdictions where it remains prohibited, appellations could provide some assurance of authenticity and ethical cultivation. They could assist the market in providing consumers with choices that meet their standards in similar fashion.

Appellations can provide consumers with more information than place of origin, as discussed earlier. The requirements common in French wine appellations (which can include restrictions on supply, eligible varietals, or alcohol content) collectively benefit the region's producers while providing information to the consumer about cultivation policies. Considering how many strains of marijuana are in existence, there would be value in a regulatory framework that easily and reliably communicates important characteristics to consumers, such as the strain and its THC levels.

In states that have legalized marijuana cultivation, many lawmakers are allowing local governments to set their own policies. This trend demonstrates that community preferences about marijuana farming are not uniform across the country. Some counties or municipalities are seeking to attract farmers and develop their own marijuana agriculture industries, while others are more cautious or restrictive in their approach. Appellations could be used in harmony with local land use and zoning decisions to satisfy these community preferences.

The prospect of a marijuana appellation system in the United States is enticing, but some tough questions need to be answered. For instance, how would appellations be enforced if the U.S. appellation system is regulated at the federal level?

Marijuana appellations would benefit from a broadly inclusive (i.e., transboundary) regulatory framework in order to maximize the impact of origin designations. The U.S. wine industry's appellations—American Viticultural Areas (AVAs)—are regulated by the federal TTB,[43] but the TTB won't be establishing a national appellation system for marijuana if cultivation remains illegal under federal law.

States can develop their own appellation frameworks, however, and as long as states maintain bans on importing and exporting marijuana, the federal government may choose not to interfere. State appellation regulations may even prove resilient if the federal prohibition is lifted and a federal agency regulates the industry.[44] Nonetheless, it will be difficult for individual counties or local governments to enforce their own appellation designations if other jurisdictions do not follow suit. Enforcement of geographic indicators outside of a regulatory body's jurisdiction is notoriously difficult. In one infamous case, it took fourteen years and a trade mission for the Napa Valley Vintners Association to convince the Chinese government to grant protected status to the term "Napa."[45]

While the marijuana industry is increasingly mobilized and represented through interest groups,[46] it will be difficult to force jurisdictions to recognize geographic indicators without the assistance of a broader regulatory framework. Still, local attempts to create appellations can generate momentum and set precedent for other jurisdictions to replicate the model. While it's not a given that the TTB will establish marijuana appellation regulations upon legalization, state and local governments can make that outcome more likely by creating the foundations for regulation. In fact, if states and marijuana farmers succeed in establishing marijuana appellations, the TTB (or another appropriately designated federal agency) will most likely be forced to consider whether federal regulation of marijuana appellations is justified. Just as federal regulation of the wine industry led to the creation of American Viticultural Areas, so federal regulation of the marijuana industry may lead to the development of American Cannabicultural Areas.

Before the establishment of federally regulated AVAs in 1978, state and county appellation designations were the norm for the wine industry.[47] AVAs can now be used to recognize wine-growing regions defined by their geographic or environmental characteristics, instead of their political boundaries, but the state and county appellations still function as legal designations of origin.[48] Until the federal government regulates marijuana agriculture, the wine industry's transition from politically defined appellations to environmentally defined appellations provides an encouraging model for the marijuana industry to follow. States and counties shouldn't hesitate to move forward with their own marijuana appellation designations despite the lack of federal involvement.

If marijuana appellations are adopted, they will need to answer a more substantive question: Should they follow the French or American approach to appellation regulations? To recap, the American wine appellation model speaks only to geographic origin, without addressing the quality of the wine. The French appellation model, on the other hand, imposes geographic, production, and quality requirements, and only allows the appellation designation if stringent cultivation rules and regulations are followed, ensuring that the appellation's wines meet high quality standards.

When deciding which system is best for the marijuana industry, regulators should keep in mind that the French appellation model—with its stringent rules and standards—was developed over hundreds of years of viticultural experimentation and refinement.[49] More than likely, it would be premature to apply similar rules to the cultivation of marijuana in its presently nascent state. Simply recognizing that appellations are a fruitful model for marijuana agriculture, and establishing those appellations, will be challenging enough. Trying to get farmers and politicians to agree on cultivation methods and standards may be too much too soon.[50]

Nonetheless, individual appellations may benefit from establishing a limited set of cultivation requirements. One category of characteristics is proving to be especially important to marijuana consumers: indicators of sustainability. Generally speaking, many marijuana consumers are demanding products that are grown organically, or with minimal environmental impact.[51] At present, however, the marijuana industry lacks a mechanism (government-sponsored or otherwise) to certify crops that meet environmental or sustainability standards.[52] Appellations can provide certifications to farmers that meet these standards, or they can make them requirements of the appellation designation.[53]

The novelty of regulating marijuana agriculture—for both regulators and farmers—calls for tolerance of innovative and diverse approaches. The effectiveness of an enterprising appellation's certification program may lead to widespread adoption or enhance the appellation's brand in the eyes of consumers. At the moment the marijuana industry is experiencing major change and heightened uncertainty, and regions should be allowed to adopt whatever marijuana appellation system makes sense. The perfect should not be allowed to become the enemy of the good in creating marijuana appellations or enabling the system's benefits.

There are signs that marijuana appellations may be on the horizon. When California Governor Jerry Brown signed the Medical Marijuana Regulation and Safety Act (MMRSA) into law in October 2015, the bill was hailed as the first step toward putting into place a regulatory framework for marijuana agriculture.[54]

Although the state had legalized medical marijuana in 1996, there had been little to no effort to regulate the industry, particularly its many farmers.[55] The MMRSA was a step in the right direction in many ways, not least of which was to prepare for full legalization of recreational use in 2016.

The MMRSA comprehensively tasked state agencies with creating regulatory frameworks for a number of key issues facing the marijuana industry, including licensing, product tracking, labeling, pesticide use, and environmental impacts.[56] Buried deep in the text of the MMRSA is a provision that would allow the newly established Bureau of Medical Marijuana Regulation to profoundly shape the nature and direction of the marijuana industry: "The bureau may establish appellations of origin for marijuana grown in California."[57]

So far, the bureau hasn't acted on its power to establish marijuana appellations in the state of California. But even if the bureau never establishes marijuana appellations, the MMRSA already prohibits the use of California county names in the marketing, labeling, or sale of marijuana products unless the marijuana was grown in that county.[58] It will be difficult for California to enforce this provision outside its borders, but considering the size of its own marijuana farming industry, simply enforcing origin designations within the state will be a powerful first step on the journey toward adopting marijuana appellations. The MMRSA provision, although seemingly innocuous, may have far-ranging effects on the marijuana industry in the United States. As the most populous state in the Union and the most prolific marijuana producer, California is likely to dictate, or at least influence, how, where, and by whom marijuana is grown.[59]

Already, grassroots efforts are under way in California to establish local designations of origin for marijuana products.[60] In mid-June 2016, the Mendocino Appellations Project released a map showing Mendocino County, California, divided into eleven marijuana appellations.[61] Mendocino County is one of the country's largest producers of marijuana, and the appellations are based on each microregion's ecological characteristics, much as the region's wine appellations are.[62]

The founder of the map, Justin Calvino, is a Mendocino farmer who is concerned about the future of his region. "The goal of the project is to form level protections for farmers here in Mendocino County," he told me. A few years ago, Justin and a few other policy-minded marijuana farmers were looking through some wine regulations, hoping to find ideas to protect family farmers. When they stumbled on the wine appellation model, they saw its potential instantly. "It was everything," Justin said. "Like we had written it for cannabis." The map has received support from marijuana farmers, Mendocino County officials, and appellations experts, and may soon provide a model for other counties and states to replicate.[63] And if the California Bureau of Medical Marijuana Regulation chooses to establish appellations of origin for marijuana agriculture in the future, the Mendocino Appellations Project is likely to play a large role in shaping the development of state-sanctioned appellations in the region.[64]

One of the farmers in the room when Justin stumbled on the wine appellation model was Hezekiah Allen. Hezekiah's roots are in Humboldt County, and after seeing the enthusiasm that Justin's Mendocino map received, Hezekiah created an appellations map for Humboldt County.[65] Though marijuana appellations may take a while to establish themselves, grassroots efforts like these can get the process started.

Eventually governments will need to get on board as well. Humboldt County officials, for their part, appear to recognize the value of their marijuana's reputation and are working on protecting their designation of origin. In 2016, the county implemented a Proof of Origin pilot program.[66] The program provides farmers with a secure stamp to affix to the label on their products as a verifiable designation of origin. That same year, the county passed a comprehensive commercial marijuana cultivation ordinance, one of the first of its kind.[67] This ordinance addresses many of the issues facing the marijuana industry, placing limits on farm size, water, and energy use. The ordinance also created a "Humboldt Artisanal Branding" certification program for small-scale, organic marijuana farms.[68]

It isn't surprising that California's active marijuana farming community is leading the charge on this issue. But the appeal of marijuana appellations is not limited to California farming regions. A proposal to establish marijuana appellations was put forward in Oregon following passage of the state's hemp and marijuana cultivation statutes in 2014.[69] The Portland State research team's marijuana terroir experiments are being conducted with an eye toward the possibility of adopting marijuana appellations in the state.

In other states, talk of appellations may be premature, and admittedly other laws or mindsets might need to be in place before appellations can take root. Crystal Oliver, an executive board member of the Washington Cannabis Farming Council, told me the climate in their state isn't ready for appellations. "We're not ready for that conversation. [Marijuana farming] needs to be recognized as agriculture first." Fair enough. But Washington can get there eventually. And advocates like Crystal will see the appeal of appellations. "I see it as the preferred evolution of the market," she said.

However, Allen St. Pierre, the executive director of the pro-legalization National Organization for the Repeal of Marijuana Laws (NORML), embraces an unregulated approach to marijuana agriculture which may reflect an entrenched resistance to the idea of appellations. He has gone on record with his belief that Big Marijuana may be the ideal future for marijuana consumers, and his message is quite simple: "What do we want? We can get it down to four words, almost a Wal-Mart bumper sticker: 'Best product, lowest cost.'"[70] The words St. Pierre uses in this quote are revealing. The "Wal-Mart bumper sticker" is a nod to the megastore vision of the marijuana industry that Big Marijuana interests are hoping for. And the word "product" subtly alludes to the idea that marijuana is one generic product, not thousands of unique, regionally cultivated strains.

"Best product, lowest price" may be a nice sentiment. Unfortunately, it will be difficult for consumers to have it both ways. Cheap, generic marijuana will occupy a portion of the market for marijuana products, but the best products won't be coming from the producers of the lowest-priced marijuana. Instead, the best products will be produced by craft farmers cultivating high-end strains. And for those farmers to deliver the unique, high-quality, regional products that consumers want, they'll need to be protected by an appellation that gives them—and their neighbors—the exclusive right to use a designation of origin.

The Champagne riots of the early twentieth century were about more than just wine labels. France had long been marked by intense regional rivalries and conflicts. The Champagne riots, by pitting regions and their economic interests against one another, represented an existential threat to national harmony and the idea of a unified French Republic. The government was trying desperately to bring the country together. It may seem odd, then, that the solution to the riots was to create the Institut National des Appellations d'Origine (INAO), the agency tasked with creating legal divisions between France's agricultural regions.

But the narrative the government sold to the people of France was that the INAO would allow each region to distinguish itself, and, in so doing, to become a representative of France to the rest of the world. Protecting the Champagne region was necessary in order to make the world see champagne as quintessentially French. And the French system of appellations was necessary to protect the very *idea* of France. A country of regions, each unique, protected by law and, standing together, redefining the image of France.[71]

American farmers are now cultivating marijuana all over the country. Thanks to the federal prohibition, each state has been allowed to develop a unique marijuana farming identity. Those identities merit protection—the protection appellations can provide. Ironically, drawing boundaries and protecting designations of origin brought the people of France together. Perhaps appellations can do the same for the United States.

7 Sun-Grown or Diesel Dope?

American agriculture is in the grip of a technological revolution as vast and as rapid as any in history. It is a revolution, which has made the American farmer the most efficient in history. It has made his productivity the marvel and envy of every nation.

—John F. Kennedy, thirty-fifth president of the United States[1]

In August 2016, I wrote an article about the promise of marijuana appellations that appeared online in *The New Republic*.[2] The article provided an overview of the benefits an appellation system could have for marijuana farmers, while arguing that some measure of organizational stability would be needed if voters across the country passed marijuana legalization initiatives in the November 2016 elections:

Marijuana appellations are not a panacea, and it will be challenging to implement and enforce "cannabicultural" designations of origin nationwide as long as a federal marijuana prohibition is in place. But at a time when lawmakers are scrambling to put regulations in place, appellations may provide the organizational structure needed to make sure marijuana agriculture remains safe and sustainable.

The article was generally well received, but in the comments, tweets, and emails I received after the article went up, one common objection stood out. The picture I was painting of a refined family farm growing marijuana in a rustic field of plants bathing in the warm summer sun was cute, but not an accurate representation of what marijuana farming looks like. In reality, the objectors argued, marijuana growing doesn't look like farming at all. The future of the marijuana industry is indoors, in warehouses or grow rooms where every minute detail can be controlled, every environmental condition dialed in to create the most optimum possible growing environment.

Some of these comments were of the not-safe-for-work variety, but this email stood out:

> Thanks for writing the article Ryan. I know you disturbed the ignorance of some of the unaware (ignorance is not about being cognitively deficient, it's just about being unaware).
>
> I am also hoping that cannabis cultivation is limited to small farmers. I live in California and I grow cannabis indoors, aerohydroponically, in my kitchen, in a 3'X4' grow tent. Unlike growing outdoors and being limited [by] the weather, along with only growing one crop per year, I grow four crops, and control all the vital variables for optimum growth. This includes 24 hours of optimum photosynthetic active radiation (PAR) during the vegetative stage, and also includes a different optimum PAR during the twelve hour[s] of darkness during the flowering stage. I control not only the temperature of the air both during the light and dark periods, but also the temperature of the root system, the temperature of the nutrients, the humidity of the air, and am also able to triple the amount of the CO_2 during photosynthesis (which plants love, thrive on, and grow faster [with]). All of these things cannot be accomplished outdoors.
>
> Growing indoors is different than growing outdoors, and the results are different too. The dispensaries in California sell a minor amount of product that is grown outdoors. You may also not know that over nine out of ten of the last cannabis cup winners from all over the world, during the last ten years or so, are grown indoors.
>
> I like your idea of "appellations," but it's a minor market—I [love] it when my ignorance is disturbed, and I hope that you think/feel the same way about yourself.
>
> All the best to you Ryan,
>
> Gregory

Indeed, Gregory, I appreciate when my ignorance is disturbed. Of course, when I wrote the article, I was aware that a significant percentage of the farming community was growing indoors. But I didn't think it would stay that way for long. I thought it was simply a relic of the prohibition era, when indoor growing kept marijuana out of sight and out of mind for neighbors and law enforcement. Was I wrong? Is the future of marijuana farming really indoors, under the bright lights of industrial warehouses?

Indoor agriculture can be traced back to the Roman Empire in the first century CE. Tiberius Claudius Nero (r. 14 to 37 CE), an emperor of sound military and fiscal prudence, had a reclusive temperament, especially in the later years of his rule. In 26 CE, he moved to the island of Capri, in part to find solitude and respite from the political and administrative duties that surrounded him in Rome. On Capri, Tiberius indulged his hedonistic desires, and created a new Roman office: the Master of Imperial Pleasures.[3]

One of his more innocent pleasures was the cucumber. Pliny the Elder observed that "there was never a day when he was not supplied with it."[4] The cucumber, however, was not capable of harvest year-round, so Tiberius's gardeners had to get creative. The solution they came up with was to plant cucumbers in large boxes furnished with wheels and windows. The boxes could be placed outside during the day, and carted back indoors at night or during foul weather, allowing the gardeners to maintain a year-round supply of cucumbers. The improvised method kept Tiberius happy, which was likely the gardeners' most immediate concern, given the emperor's alleged and unpredictable penchant for executions, but their legacy was more enduring. They are credited with creating the first greenhouse, and with it, the advent of indoor agriculture.

It took a while for the idea to catch on. Italians built the first modern greenhouses in the thirteenth century to house the exotic plants explorers brought back from the tropics. Though prohibitively expensive for most, aristocrats in France and England commissioned the construction of large, glass-walled greenhouses to support their tastes for exotic fruits. No expense was spared in the construction of the *orangerie* at the Palace of Versailles, and Louis XIV made sure it was stocked with the world's largest collection of orange trees.[5] The aristocratic interest in exotic plants spurred a more general interest in the study of botany, prompting the world's great universities to build greenhouses designed for research and observation.

The Victorian era coincided with the golden age of the greenhouse. Taxes on window glass were repealed, paving the way for individuals to build modest greenhouses of their own, and for governments to build soaring, elaborate greenhouses for the people. These beautified greenhouses represented the Victorians' architectural and agricultural ideals, allowing ordinary citizens to interact with nature's rare species from all over the world.[6]

Early America was known for its outdoor agriculture, and the prevailing sentiment at the time—that the continent's lands and natural resources were limitless—provided little incentive for farmers to build enclosures around their crops. But greenhouses had their place on the plantations of the wealthy. George Washington built a greenhouse to grow pineapples for his guests. And Frederick Douglass, African-American statesman and abolitionist, was a child slave on a plantation that contained a greenhouse for oranges and agricultural experiments.[7]

Technological advances in the twentieth century brought the greenhouse to the masses. Affordable polyethylene plastic film could replace more expensive glass, and with less mass weighing down the structure, cheap metals or PVC tubing could be used for support. While rudimentary, these alternatives made it possible for small-scale gardeners and horticulturalists to build their own greenhouses.

Once electricity generation and transmission became widely available, the commercial potential of indoor agriculture could be realized on a larger scale. The key ingredients to a thriving greenhouse operation are ventilation (which keeps air moving and regulates temperature and humidity) and heating (which keeps plants from freezing and also regulates temperature). Both ingredients require energy, electricity being the most common source. A third ingredient is an elevated level of carbon dioxide to enrich the greenhouse's atmosphere, thereby stimulating plant growth. Most commonly this elevated level is achieved by burning CO_2-emitting fossil fuels in a generator.[8] Commercial-scale generator technology made carbon dioxide enrichment possible and profitable.[9]

The world leader in commercial greenhouse agriculture is, indisputably, the Netherlands. Despite being a small, densely populated country without much land to spare for large-scale farming, the Netherlands has become the world's second largest food exporter by value.[10] Deliberate investment in greenhouse technology and indoor crop production has made this possible.

The Dutch countryside is littered with sprawling greenhouse complexes, each one closely controlling growing conditions to maximize productivity. The Netherlands has some of the highest crop yields in the world, producing more tomatoes, green peppers, and cucumbers per square mile than any other country.[11] Dutch flower producers dominate the global flower trade, claiming a 44 percent market share.[12] They, too, capitalize on greenhouse technology. And many of these greenhouse operations aren't run by agribusiness conglomerates but by thousands of family farms. By harnessing the power of indoor agriculture, the Netherlands have become an unlikely agricultural powerhouse.[13]

In the twenty-first century, indoor agriculture is receiving renewed attention as public- and private-sector interests alike look for solutions to the world's growing food supply and sustainability challenges. The United

Nations Population Division estimates that the human population of 7.6 billion will rise to nearly 10 billion by 2050.[14] To feed a population that large, the U.N.'s Food and Agriculture Organization estimates that agricultural production will need to rise by at least 50 percent.[15]

It's not clear how a 50 percent increase in food production will be achieved. Half of the world's habitable land—and 70 percent of available water supplies—are already dedicated to agriculture.[16] The agriculture industry might be able to find marginally more land and water,[17] but at what cost? Unsustainable farming practices have already created unprecedented deforestation, desertification, soil degradation, and water pollution problems worldwide. And climate change (which agriculture is partly responsible for creating) adds uncertainty, as long-held assumptions about the resources and environmental conditions available to agriculture need to be questioned.

Given these constraints, the only solution left seems to be to increase yields—in other words, to make more with less. In the past, agricultural production increases have been heavily dependent on yield growth.[18] However, the growth rate of yields has been falling in recent years, stoking fears that food production will not be capable of meeting a rise in demand.[19] Many of the reliable yield-increasing innovations of the past—genetic modifications, fertilizers, and pesticides—are no longer popular options for environmentally minded countries, either. When it comes to sustainably feeding a growing population, there are no easy answers.[20]

In this context, futuristic entrepreneurs and investment firms are probing for new approaches to food production, and no idea is off the table. Recent innovations include everything from GPS-connected tractors to drone surveillance to microbe-based products. The desire to produce food in or near urban centers (to reduce transportation costs and impacts) has led to widespread adoption of rooftop gardens and inner-city farming collectives, or community-supported agriculture programs that support local family farms in periurban areas.

A major source of innovation is coming from the marriage of agriculture and information technology. Dubbed "smart farming" (or precision farming), the underlying idea is that a computer program or farm management system can monitor growth conditions (such as the climate, water supply, soil quality, and disease vulnerability) and, in many cases, make changes to those conditions automatically, in real time. Essentially, Big

Data technologies are being harnessed to increase agricultural productivity. The usual agribusiness giants are involved, but the emphasis on computing software and the potential for disruption has naturally attracted tech start-ups and Silicon Valley moguls as well.[21]

A controlled indoor environment is the perfect place for these trends in urban agriculture and precision farming to meet. Indoor farms can be located almost anywhere, including urban industrial zones, because computers monitor and control the environment using precision farming technologies. Recently, indoor farms have begun to move away from the greenhouse model, favoring windowless warehouses or shipping containers in which every growing condition is artificially recreated—including light. "Vertical farming," as it's called, is a form of indoor agriculture in which crops are stacked on top of each other. Plants may be potted in soil, placed in water (known as hydroponics), or have their root system suspended in the air (known as aeroponics). Either way, artificial lights allow the plants to be grown year-round, at whatever light intensity and duration the farmer desires. The heating, ventilation, and irrigation systems can all be monitored and controlled from a computer, and smart farming software can make horticultural decisions without the assistance of a human farmer.

In 2010, no commercial vertical farms existed anywhere in the United States. By 2017, vertical farms were up and running in Detroit, Houston, New York City, and Seattle.[22] Chicago has emerged as the country's hub for vertical farming, with several well-funded, large-scale indoor operations in the metropolitan area.[23] One study estimates the market value of vertical farming will reach $4 billion by 2020. By then the precision farming software market is expected to reach nearly $2 billion as well.[24]

The advantages of vertical farming are numerous. As mentioned earlier, the farms can be located in or near cities, reducing transportation costs and providing fresher produce to consumers. Vertical farms can be set at exact specifications to produce optimum growing conditions, and those conditions plus the use of artificial lighting and year-round cultivation have dramatically increased yields per square foot. By increasing yields and providing alternative food sources, vertical farms may reduce the need to expand outdoor farming's footprint and environmental impacts.

The disadvantages may be equally numerous, however. Assuming vertical farms can be profitable (they are only feasible due to a recent drop in the cost of artificial lights), the energy resources needed to replicate the sun's light energy will always be significant. At some point solar panels may be able to provide those resources, but for the moment the energy demands of vertical farms outstrip solar capabilities, such that indoor farms are still burning up fossil fuels and electricity to power their lighting, heating, irrigation, and ventilation systems. Those vertical farms that enrich their atmospheres with elevated levels of carbon dioxide burn even more fuel. And finally, vertical farms will need to find ways to minimize light and water pollution.[25] All these costs result in produce that is pricey and thus inaccessible to many consumers.

Though the Netherlands has proved the viability of large-scale greenhouse agriculture, it is too soon to tell if completely artificial indoor environments are capable of producing meaningful crop yields while remaining financially and environmentally sustainable. Vertical farms have nevertheless captured the attention and imagination of venture capitalists and start-up investors, who are pouring more money into them every year. The promise of a controlled agricultural environment is intoxicating for many visionaries. A century from now, we may look back and wonder why we didn't start farming indoors sooner—or vertical farms may be nothing more than a passing fad, with flaws so obvious we'll wonder why anyone even tried.

Of course, if vertical farmers are looking for encouragement or inspiration, they need look no further than the marijuana industry. During the prohibition era, indoor growing was not only feasible for growers, it was also wildly profitable. These growers pioneered many contemporary indoor farming methods, at great risk to themselves and their families.

Dave Smiles, whose vertical farming operation in Florida is one of the largest in the United States, understands the legacy these marijuana growers are leaving behind: "If it wasn't for underground illicit agriculture, the technology wouldn't be there. It's on the shoulders of all those who have been incarcerated that now growing food indoors is viable."[26] But as marijuana agriculture transitions away from its illicit roots, will growing marijuana indoors remain viable?

When the Reagan administration raised the stakes of marijuana farming in the 1980s, its goal was to reduce the supply of marijuana in the United States by eradicating plants, increasing minimum penalties for drug crimes, incarcerating growers, and dissuading would-be growers from jumping into the market. The shock-and-awe tactics employed by militarized drug enforcement authorities succeeded in driving out some growers, like Elaine, who had other interests or sources of income. But most growers simply adjusted to the new realities of the war on drugs. Those who kept their crops outside diversified, maintaining several smaller plots instead of one large one. Many others adapted to the aerial assaults by moving their growing operations indoors.

Once inside, growers closed themselves off to the outside world. Plants were grown in warehouses, basements, closets, spare bedrooms, storage sheds, shipping containers, garages, and attics. Indoor grows had the advantage of being private and harder to detect by aerial and terrestrial surveillance. Plus, it's trickier for law enforcement to barge in on a private enclosure without a warrant. Growers in some parts of the country had already started growing indoors, lacking the ideal outdoor growing conditions and rugged solitude that blessed farmers in northern California.

From a productivity standpoint, the transition during the Reagan administration was hit and miss at first. The agriculture industry had not developed the twenty-first-century smart farming technologies that make indoor cultivation the highly sophisticated and productive practice it is today. Artificial lights were rudimentary and expensive. Ventilation equipment wasn't designed to eliminate odors before blowing air outside. Carbon dioxide enrichment was not widespread. Strains had not been bred to grow productively in small enclosures.

But marijuana farmers are a resilient bunch, and the profitability of illicit marijuana sparked dramatic gains in productivity. Growers adopted the best practices and growing methods used by professional greenhouses, including hydroponics, aeroponics, and carbon dioxide enrichment. Lighting, heating, irrigation, and ventilation systems were modified to create and maintain intense and highly productive growing conditions. The domestic indoor marijuana farming demographic was large enough that eventually horticulture equipment manufacturers started marketing products tailored to the marijuana industry. Indoor growers became proficient in replicating the life-inducing gifts of Mother Nature. In some ways, they were able to create growing environments that were even more optimized for plant growth than the natural environment in their region.

Best of all, breeders were able to propagate strains that thrived indoors. Indica strains—being characteristically short, bushy, and quick to flower—provided an ideal starting point.[27] They fit easily into enclosed spaces, and a lighting system could be timed to manipulate the plants into flowering even earlier than usual. Over time, hybrid strains were fine-tuned to the point that they produced plants with these characteristics in the extreme: indoor strains became very short, very potent, very quick to flower, and very high-yielding.

Indoor grows also retained a key advantage over their outdoor competitors: they could grow year-round. Whereas an outdoor farm can only cultivate plants from the spring planting season to the fall harvest, an indoor farm is oblivious to the changing seasons and can continue growing crop after crop after crop indefinitely. This fact, combined with advances in growing methods and marijuana genetics, convinced many farmers that indoor cultivation represented the superior agricultural approach. Throw in the privacy and security advantages, and it was a no-brainer. Northern California could keep its outdoor farms; the rest of the country would be growing inside.

Yet outdoor farms—especially those in the Emerald Triangle—kept their footing in the marijuana industry. After all, it remained much easier to grow in wide open spaces where plants can grow larger and more numerous. But as the era of legalization dawned and consumers started buying in dispensaries instead of on the street, many developed a taste for the potent, consistent buds produced indoors. This preference started to be reflected in the economics of marijuana agriculture—indoor growers started receiving (and still receive) more for their product than outdoor growers.

When they picture vast warehouses filled with thousands of plants being cultivated by modern farm management software, many entrepreneurs believe they're seeing the future of the marijuana industry. And they may be. But the prohibition era smoothed over some of the most crippling disadvantages of growing marijuana indoors. It may be possible, perhaps even likely, for indoor farms to survive. But it won't be as easy as it may seem today.

The most problematic variable of an indoor marijuana farm is the same variable that is problematic for other indoor farming operations. The godlike ability to control and manipulate every detail of the environment is extraordinary—but it's also very expensive. The cost of running high-intensity artificial lights year-round is unique to indoor grows, for starters. Outdoor farms, of course, get their light energy free from the sun. A modern indoor facility, outfitted with modern equipment and technology, is also a major investment. In the prohibition era, marijuana prices were inflated to the point that many inefficiencies were overlooked. Now that prices have plummeted, the production costs of indoor farming may not remain viable.

Compared to outdoor farms, indoor farms have much higher start-up and operating costs. According to a 2017 estimate, the typical start-up costs for an indoor facility with 10,000 square feet of plant canopy totaled roughly $750,000. Annual operating costs for the same facility were nearly $1.3 million.[28] Those costs are offset by higher revenues—indoor grows can harvest year-round, and indoor marijuana fetches the highest prices on the market. But the high start-up and operating costs are a barrier to entry for many small-scale farmers, and it's not clear if indoor marijuana will continue to receive the higher prices necessary to offset these production costs.

Of course, the figures above are only estimates, and in an industry still operating in a legal gray area, accurate estimates are notoriously elusive. In addition, the single largest operating cost for an indoor farm is the cost of its energy use, which in the United States varies widely by location. In 2018, Washington State had the lowest industrial electricity costs in the nation, at under 5 cents/kWh. Electricity costs were almost five times more expensive in Hawaii, the most expensive state, at nearly 25 cents/kWh.[29] For indoor farms operating off the grid, the cost of running a diesel generator is substantial as well (and gives rise to the pejorative term "diesel dope"). The financial viability of an indoor facility will thus be heavily dependent on its location. In California (11.5 cents/kWh), indoor production costs may be prohibitive, especially when faced with competition from the state's resolute outdoor farming community. But in Washington or Oregon (5.9 cents/kWh), electricity is relatively cheap and may support an indoor farming sector.

Outdoor marijuana cultivation has the advantage of completely avoiding the energy costs of reproducing nature's elements—and outdoor farms don't need a pricey facility, either. The start-up and operating costs of an outdoor farm are therefore much lower. To start an outdoor farm with 50,000 square feet of plant canopy (five times the size of the indoor facility described above) costs only $500,000, and the annual operating costs are similarly modest—roughly $830,000.[30] Revenues tend to be lower as well, however, since "sun-grown" marijuana—reflective of nature's inconsistencies—isn't as well received by consumers. But at a time when prices are falling drastically, the lower production costs of outdoor farms may enable farmers to withstand more risk.

Outdoor farms are attractive for other reasons as well. For connoisseurs or purists, the terroir will come through in marijuana grown in a natural environment. Obviously, the terroir of an indoor operation will not be associated with a geographic location or farming community. Environmentalists may also appreciate the organic potential of outdoor farms; it is still difficult for indoor farmers to grow plants so intensively without the assistance of chemical fertilizers or pesticides. As the industry matures and marijuana tourism becomes a new source of income, outdoor farms could become a more attractive destination, much as vineyards have capitalized on the rustic ideals of their patrons.

And while indoor farmers are uniquely positioned to grow strains bred for indoor cultivation, outdoor farmers have their own gamut of strains to choose from. Sativa strains, for example, which grow tall, slender, high-yielding plants, take longer to flower, but outdoor farms have the time and space for these plants to reach their full potential.

An oft-cited downside of outdoor farms is that they are limited to producing one crop cycle per year. But this is a misconception. It's true that indoor farms have an advantage because they can manipulate the photoperiods provided by their lighting systems. This allows them to trick plants into thinking the "days" are going by faster than they really are, hastening the arrival of the fall flowering season. But outdoor farms employ a similar method called light deprivation ("light dep" for short). A basic light dep can be constructed by installing several plastic or metal arches over a plot of sun-grown marijuana plants. To trick the plants into thinking the fall flowering season is arriving, the photoperiods are manipulated by pulling a blackout tarp over the arches in the early evening, often around 6 p.m.

Instead of waiting the whole summer to harvest marijuana, farmers with a light dep can harvest plants in two months. Depending on the weather and a farmer's level of motivation, that means a light dep can produce two to three crop cycles per year, a nice complement to the crops grown all summer long. Light deps are labor-intensive, and were disfavored when prices were high during the prohibition era. Now that competition is fiercer, light deps have become a common sight on outdoor farms, so much so that 6 p.m.—when farmers all over the Emerald Triangle hurry back to their deps to tarp—is jokingly referred to as "Humboldt Rush Hour."

While light deps minimize the seasonal limitations of outdoor farming, they can't eliminate them completely. Mother Nature provides free light energy, favorable climates, and healthy soils. But in outdoor marijuana farming, you take the good with the bad. In the early autumn of 2016, the bad came in the form of northern California getting slammed with unseasonably early rains. Without knowing when the rains would let up, farmers were forced to make a risky decision: either harvest what they could (and make peace with the low yields), or wait out the rains and hope the crops weren't ruined by mold or mildew. Jack chose the former, and he was glad he did. His yields were disappointing, but some friends in the community who waited for a change in the weather lost entire crops to mold. The following season, in 2017, an unusually snowy winter delayed the start of the growing season. With snow still on the ground well into spring, crops were planted later than planned. Jack had hoped to light dep his way to three crop cycles that summer, but the delayed start made him settle for two.

Indoor versus outdoor farming is a matter of fierce debate in the marijuana farming community. There is, however, a middle ground. Many states with legal markets are issuing permits for "mixed light" cultivation, which essentially means greenhouse cultivation. Greenhouses represent a compromise on virtually every tradeoff discussed above. By harnessing the sun's light energy, costs are lower than purely indoor operations, yet the enclosed structure can still be controlled to create optimum growing conditions. Both production costs and revenues are higher than those of outdoor farms but lower than those of indoor farms. And like the other methods, the financial picture can vary widely depending on the size and sophistication of the operation. A greenhouse can be a small, rudimentary structure designed to supplement a larger operation, or a large, modern greenhouse can be the entire operation.

The question I'd like an answer to is, which of these approaches—indoor, outdoor, or mixed—represents the future of marijuana agriculture? For more than three years, I've been asking this question of people in the industry, including farmers, retailers, advocates, academics, and policymakers. The (unscientific) results don't paint a clear picture.

Many respondents envision a future in which all three methods coexist. For this group, indoor and outdoor farming communities have come too far for either demographic to simply fade away. As illustrated by the variance in electricity costs, some regions of the country may come to favor one approach, while other regions favor another. Or farmers will start to incorporate all three elements into their business models. Jack, for example, is primarily an outdoor farmer, but his barn supports an indoor nursery, while his greenhouse readies clones and starts for planting in the spring.

The second group of respondents is more skeptical of the economics of indoor farming; they can't see how the energy costs of indoor agriculture will be feasible in the long term. This group believes that outdoor farmers will be able to match the quality of indoor marijuana before indoor farmers can match the production costs of outdoor farms. If large-scale outdoor farms start producing massive quantities of marijuana, driving prices down, indoor growers will be forced to cater to a small high-end market. At the same time, if craft outdoor growers are producing organic marijuana with terroir, the connoisseur crowd might not have a need for indoor marijuana.

A third group sees the landscape in more political terms. Because the marijuana industry is highly regulated in legal markets, they believe farmers may adopt growing methods or practices as a result of political decrees. If so, indoor farms stand to benefit. Many politicians—forced to deal with the nuts and bolts of legalization after a voter-led ballot initiative—are happy to adopt policies that keep the marijuana industry hidden from view. From a visual perspective, indoor farms are the most discreet. If they keep their odors and light pollution in check, many indoor farms look like any other nondescript warehouse, offensive to virtually no one. Greenhouses and outdoor farms are less secure, subjecting unsuspecting passersby to their unsavory contents.

There is already evidence that the third group is correct. Many states or local jurisdictions have adopted regulations or ordinances requiring that marijuana agriculture take place indoors. Colorado imposes enclosure and security requirements, for example, and New York and Florida have issued cultivation licenses only to indoor growing facilities. Canada's national medical marijuana laws do not allow for commercial outdoor cultivation. Family farming advocates in Washington are fighting to preserve their right to farm outside, under threat from lawmakers and energy lobbyists intent on ushering the farming community indoors.

It is unfortunate, in my view, that politicians won't give outdoor farms a chance. Land use and zoning laws could still expel outdoor farms to rural locales, and cultivation regulations can address whatever security concerns may exist. But a blanket ban on outdoor cultivation is a draconian imposition on the legal marijuana market at a time when the industry is still trying to find its identity. Perhaps I'm biased, having friends in northern California's outdoor growing community. But a future in which farmers aren't free to grow a legal crop on American soil is not a future I'm interested in.

Jack had a good laugh when I showed him Gregory's email in response to my *New Republic* article. "Indoor growers have a hell of a superiority complex," he told me. "But I mean that with lots of love."

Indoor marijuana farms may be more expensive to operate, but they justify those costs by producing quality marijuana that currently fetches the highest prices on the market. The way Jack sees it, if these indoor grows survive in the long term, that means there's a reliable market for high-end, expensive product. And that's a great thing for all craft farmers, regardless of their agricultural loyalties. If consumers will pay for the potent, consistent marijuana produced by indoor growers, they might be willing to pay more for organic, family-farmed sun-grown marijuana with terroir, too.

"If indoor stays alive, that means people love great buds enough to not just choose shitty brick," Jack said. "So let's hope this dude is right."

8 A Strain on the Environment

We have to see clearly that whatever destroys the forest, except to make way for agriculture, threatens our well-being.
—Theodore Roosevelt, twenty-sixth president of the United States

The nation that destroys its soil destroys itself.
—Franklin D. Roosevelt, thirty-second president of the United States[1]

All of this might seem diabolical, but the saloon-keeper was in no wise to blame for it. He was in the same plight as the manufacturer who has to adulterate and misrepresent his product. If he does not, someone else will.
—Upton Sinclair, *The Jungle*, 1906[2]

I'll admit I had doubts when Jack told me he was planning to buy a farm. He had the talent to succeed as a farmer and businessman, I knew that. And he assured me that the property—which included vineyards, a winery, and several living cabins, all located in a desirable location near the Klamath River—had long-term potential. Even if the market soured on craft weed, the farm figured to hold most of its value.

But it wasn't the business plan I was worried about. When Jack bought the farm in 2015, marijuana farmers were still in legal limbo. The Obama administration had relaxed the federal government's stance toward prohibition, which provided some comfort. A 2013 memo from the Department of Justice instructed U.S. Attorneys not to prosecute individuals who were in compliance with state marijuana laws.[3] The memo outlined some egregious activities that would warrant federal attention, but a small-scale grow on private land wasn't on the list. Nonetheless, a presidential election was only a year away, and it was hard to tell what position a new administration might take on marijuana prohibition.

California marijuana politics were hard to read as well. Although medical marijuana cultivation had been legal in California since 1996, nineteen years later the state had yet to put any kind of agricultural regulations in place. Farmers were trying to cover their bases by collecting medical marijuana cards that might, in theory, allow them to grow plants on behalf of card holders. But it wasn't clear whether there was an upper limit on the number of plants that could be grown, and the state hadn't issued—or even created—cultivation licenses that could reassure farmers they were in compliance. Without a regulatory framework in place, it was hard to know if Jack's farm was a risky investment.

To make matters worse, the reputation of the outdoor farming community in northern California was taking a hit. In 2014, the governor of California had issued a drought state of emergency in response to ongoing shortfalls in freshwater supplies.[4] The declaration asked state agencies and officials to "take all necessary actions to prepare for these drought conditions."[5] The drought in California and across the United States had become a mainstream topic of conversation, dominating headlines and forcing governments to reexamine their water regulations. As a result, California's state agencies were gearing up to take a second look at the marijuana industry.

Around the same time, *Mother Jones* magazine published an article entitled "The Landscape-Scarring, Energy-Sucking, Wildlife-Killing Reality of Pot Farming."[6] As the title suggests, the article brought to light the most severe environmental impacts of marijuana agriculture, including pesticide and rodenticide pollution, illegal water withdrawals, soil erosion, and energy use. Much of the anecdotal evidence was connected to illegal trespass grows, but the whole farming community was implicated.

Then, in 2015, the first scientific study of the impacts of marijuana cultivation on water resources was published. Data was taken from the Eel River watershed in Humboldt County, not too far from Jack's farm. The research team, led by California Department of Fish and Wildlife employees, looked at satellite imagery to estimate the number of marijuana plants being grown in the watershed, then compared the water needs of those plants with historical flow data from the Eel River. The researchers found that the marijuana industry's demand for water often outstripped water supplies completely, leaving streambeds dry and endangered species like the coho salmon without a suitable habitat.[7]

In late June 2015, a few months after Jack had moved onto the farm, a convoy of vehicles carrying enforcement officers from four different counties of northern California drove up the remote and rugged slopes of Island Mountain.[8] (The mountain had been given its name by early settlers who observed that it was nearly surrounded by the waters of the Eel River and its tributaries.)[9] The enforcement officers conducted open-field searches on private lands, and by the end of the weeklong Operation Emerald Tri-County, they had confiscated 86,578 marijuana plants.[10]

While police raids of marijuana farms is nothing new for the Emerald Triangle, this particular operation raised some eyebrows. Unusually for a raid of this magnitude, no federal officials were involved—the raid was a wholly state-run operation.[11] Also unusual were the lands targeted by the raid. At that point, most marijuana plants seized by law enforcement were being grown illegally on public lands, but this operation went after privately held marijuana grows with some measure of legal protection under the state's Compassionate Use Act.

Though the raid signaled a shift in the enforcement of marijuana laws, it was not because the counties were cracking down on marijuana per se. The enforcement officers were joined, not by federal officials, but by personnel from the California Department of Fish and Wildlife.[12] The counties claimed the raid was motivated by violations of state water regulations, not by the fact that marijuana was being cultivated.[13] After finding unpermitted stream bed alterations, diversions, and reservoirs, the officials confiscated the privately grown plants.[14]

The environmental intentions of the state may not have produced the greenest long-term consequences, however. Several targets of the raids were members of a political action group working with the counties to draft ordinances that would increase transparency and bring growers into compliance with environmental laws.[15] The group's director expressed dismay that the raid would force growers back into the shadows, away from the state's regulatory framework.[16] A previous effort in 2010 had been successful in partnering private growers with county officials to monitor plants and facilitate regulatory compliance, but a federal raid and subpoena of the program's paperwork shut it down and broke up the partnership in 2012.[17] The community feared Operation Emerald Tri-County would do the same, wasting years of delicate negotiations.

The environmental impacts of marijuana agriculture continue to attract the public's attention, and for good reason: any type of agriculture, left unchecked, has the potential to negatively impact the environment. Marijuana is no exception. But what frustrates many in the marijuana farming community is that some states haven't acknowledged that marijuana is a crop in the first place. Without that prerequisite, how can anyone hope to address environmental impacts?

Crystal and Kevin Oliver, outdoor farmers and marijuana legalization advocates in Washington State, organized a grassroots campaign against a proposal to classify marijuana farming as a "moderate-hazard factory industrial use." The classification would have forced farmers to grow indoors. Their local campaign was successful, but the same dynamic is repeating itself all over the state. Spokane County commissioners drafted language excluding marijuana farming as an agricultural activity for zoning purposes, and state regulators are hesitant to classify marijuana farming as agriculture lest it provide tax breaks to marijuana farmers. "We're fighting for our right to farm," Crystal told me with exasperation. "They're telling us we're not farmers."

In New York, the approach has been similarly dismissive of the agricultural sector of the marijuana industry. In 2014 the state passed the Compassionate Care Act legalizing medicinal marijuana.[18] But the law as written rejects the concept of marijuana agriculture altogether, referring to the process of growing marijuana plants as "manufacturing."[19] To the extent the law addresses marijuana "manufacturing" at all, it requires that plants be grown indoors.[20]

For twenty years after California became the first state to legalize medicinal marijuana, laws focused mainly on regulating physicians, patients, and dispensaries. The state acted as if marijuana appeared out of thin air. Or perhaps the state's regulatory priorities considered that marijuana agriculture did not need regulation.

In Colorado, a task force established to propose legislative and executive actions after voters legalized recreational marijuana use in 2012 identified some agricultural issues—such as regulating pesticides, taxing cultivators, and establishing cultivation limits—but broader issues central to agricultural development (such as water use or permitted cultivation practices) were not addressed.[21] Two years later, the Colorado Department of Agriculture was still paralyzed by this definitional dilemma. "For food crops, a tolerance (of pesticide residues) must be established. No tolerances have been established for marijuana because they are not recognized as a legal 'agricultural crop,'" the agency said.[22]

The point is that in many states farmers don't have any agricultural regulations to comply with. And in an unregulated environment, it is unsurprising that some farmers are taking extreme measures to stay competitive.

States are free to call marijuana farming whatever they want, of course. But their terminology of choice won't change the fact that marijuana farmers are cultivating crops for commercial purposes—the very definition of "agriculture." Unfortunately, until states accept marijuana cultivation as an agricultural activity, farmers will not be regulated, a shortcoming that may be most problematic for the environment. Marijuana agriculture creates environmental risks and impacts that could be minimized with laws and regulations. At the moment, however, farmers are still waiting to see them.

Sensitivity to water shortages in northern California raised a red flag right as Jack was mulling over the purchase of the farm, the biggest decision of his life. Fortunately, the deed to his farm included water rights he could use for agricultural and domestic purposes, and his farming methods are admirably sustainable. He moved forward with the acquisition, and hasn't looked back.

Nonetheless, once I started researching the relationship between marijuana farming and state water laws, I realized there weren't any clear guidelines for marijuana farmers. Marijuana plants require significant quantities of water resources, and existing water laws might not be capable of accommodating the marijuana industry.

In the American West, the prior appropriation doctrine still forms the basis for most state water law frameworks. The prior appropriation doctrine allocates water according to a priority system, with the oldest (or "senior") water rights holders getting first dibs, while junior rights holders get whatever is left over. In prior appropriation states, regulators have tough choices to make. If they don't give water rights to marijuana farmers, those farmers will either make illegal appropriations to maintain their operation or move their operation out of state. If regulators do issue water rights, they may be affecting existing appropriative rights that give priority to senior rights holders.[23]

Fortunately, most prior appropriation states administer water rights through a regulatory agency that could address water rights for marijuana farmers proactively, without significantly interfering with existing rights.

While the prior appropriation doctrine will make it challenging to appease a brand-new agricultural subsector, states have more flexibility than a strict legal interpretation would suggest.

The federal Bureau of Reclamation complicates matters considerably, however. The Bureau operates in only seventeen states in the American West, but is nonetheless the largest wholesale water supplier in the United States.[24] It provides irrigation water to one-fifth of western farmers, and supplies municipal, residential, and industrial water to 31 million people.[25] The Bureau of Reclamation has not been cooperative with states that have legalized marijuana cultivation. In May 2014, the Bureau announced that it would not allow water supplies or facilities it controls to be used for purposes of cultivating marijuana.[26] That includes the 475 dams, 337 reservoirs, and 8,116 miles of irrigation canals it controls, and the water those facilities supply.[27] The prohibition has confused water rights holders throughout prior appropriation jurisdictions.

The Bureau of Reclamation provides water to two-thirds of the irrigated land in Washington, for example, a state where recreational and medicinal marijuana cultivation has been legal since 2012.[28] But it's not clear how farmers growing multiple crops on those lands would be regulated if one of those crops is marijuana. As one state manager for the Roza Irrigation District put it, "these kinds of details have not been fleshed out."[29] The state's regulatory agency with primary jurisdiction over marijuana claims that it would be impossible to determine how many marijuana farmers are using Bureau of Reclamation waters.[30]

The Bureau of Reclamation provides water to even more lands in Colorado,[31] where regulators are similarly confused. One water supplier insisted that its water supplies could not be interfered with by federal officials despite having to pass through a Bureau of Reclamation dam facility.[32] By contrast, a water district in the same area imposed a moratorium on marijuana irrigation in order to comply with the federal policy, before lifting the moratorium in spite of the policy.[33]

States east of the Mississippi River should have a slightly easier time adjusting to the legal marijuana industry. The water laws of eastern states are governed by the doctrine of riparianism, in which riparian water rights are not fixed but accommodate reasonable uses of shared waters.[34] If states classify marijuana farming as agriculture, irrigating a marijuana crop will likely be considered a reasonable use of water (agricultural uses have traditionally been recognized as a reasonable use of water in these states).

Like their western counterparts, many eastern states now use riparian principles to inform a more regulated and proactive water rights regime, issuing water use permits that can expire or be revoked depending on water supplies. These states may not have as much flexibility in the short term if existing permits allocate all of the available water resources, but in the long term, agencies will retain the flexibility to shape water use in the states by controlling the permit process.[35] This flexibility should provide ample room to maneuver in the new marijuana economy.

In many states, the challenges of regulating water use on marijuana farms remain theoretical, but in states like California the issue is very real. Water is already a scarce and fiercely controlled resource, with a complex system of riparian, appropriative, and groundwater rights.[36] The various water rights regimes provide multiple opportunities to create or recognize rights to water for marijuana farmers, but the complexity of the system will make it challenging to capitalize on those opportunities. California's decentralized approach to marijuana regulation, meanwhile, is allowing local governments to move in many different directions, sometimes at cross purposes.[37]

Two themes emerged from my research on water law and marijuana farming. In theory, while old-school doctrines of water law are often criticized for being rigid and antiquated, the law has enough flexibility for regulators to provide water to marijuana farmers without significantly disrupting existing water rights. This is particularly true in jurisdictions that adopt a modified or regulatory version of traditional doctrines.

In practice, however, the initial signs coming from states where marijuana cultivation is legal suggest that the theoretical ability of water law doctrine to incorporate marijuana cultivation is not sufficient to ensure a smooth transition. There are too many legal ambiguities in both water laws and marijuana laws for the simultaneous application of both to be able to function coherently and consistently. In order to promote sustainable, responsible, and legal marijuana cultivation, while also administering water rights equitably, states will need to adjust their regulatory frameworks to address the challenges that marijuana legalization presents.

There are reasons to be optimistic. California's Medical Marijuana Regulation and Safety Act (MMRSA) and Adult Use of Marijuana Act (AUMA) of 2016 both contain ambitious proposals to create comprehensive regulations for marijuana agriculture, including water allocation provisions.[38] A variety of state agencies have been granted new powers to regulate the environmental impacts of marijuana farming, including the Department of Food and Agriculture, Department of Fish and Wildlife, Department of Public Health, and the State Water Resources Control Board.[39] It remains to be seen if these agencies will be able to coordinate, articulate, and enforce clear policies. Still, the laws are a promising sign that states are beginning to take water resource issues seriously.

From a hydrological perspective, to draw a distinction between water quantity and water quality is illogical: when water levels drop, water quality often deteriorates as pollutants become less diluted. Conversely, when pollutants are introduced into a water resource, the quantity of clean water available is reduced. Nevertheless, modern water law systems do, for the most part, distinguish between water quantity and water quality, with some regulations addressing water allocations and others addressing water pollution. Just as water allocation laws will need to reconcile tensions between marijuana agriculture and water rights, so too will water quality laws need to reconcile marijuana agriculture's impacts on water quality. And although research on the topic remains limited, what studies do exist suggest that if left unchecked, marijuana agriculture may have significant negative impacts on water quality.

A 2013 study on wildlife mortality found a link between rodenticides found in dead mammals and the density of nearby marijuana farms, suggesting that pesticides and fertilizers may be seeping into the broader environment, including water resources.[40] And the deforestation, land terracing, and road building associated with large marijuana grows contribute to erosion and sediment loading of streams, according to a 2011 study of western public lands.[41]

More research is needed, but there is sufficient evidence to conclude that marijuana agriculture produces the same three forms of runoff pollution (pesticides, fertilizers, and sediment) that have been a problem for agricultural regulation in general. For this reason, states might need to reconsider their existing water quality regulations to address runoff pollution from marijuana farms.

One major difference between water allocation laws and water quality laws is that water allocation has traditionally been a state function, whereas the federal government has stepped in to regulate water quality through enactment and enforcement of the Clean Water Act (CWA).[42] The CWA declared it the policy of Congress to "recognize, preserve, and protect the primary responsibilities and rights of States to prevent, reduce, and eliminate pollution."[43] To implement this objective, Congress uses financial incentives and the threat of preemption to obtain state participation and compliance with the Act.

For example, states are allowed to create their own water pollution control plans, including state water quality standards, effluent limitations, and watercourse-specific designated uses.[44] If the state fails to do so, or if its standards do not meet federal minimums,[45] the Environmental Protection Agency (EPA) is authorized to regulate on behalf of the state.[46] This rarely happens, in part because Congress provides funding for the development of pollution control programs,[47] research,[48] and construction of treatment works,[49] a major incentive for state participation.

Unfortunately, the Clean Water Act has not been effective at eliminating pollution from agricultural runoff, largely because the CWA is not designed to do so.[50] Instead of regulating agricultural runoff directly, states and the federal government attempt to regulate runoff indirectly by funding pollution control programs that enhance monitoring or encourage sustainable farming practices.[51] These collaborative programs often involve a diverse set of stakeholders that include state and federal agencies, and representatives of the agricultural industry.[52]

Approaches that encourage stakeholder engagement and provide incentives for farmers to participate are precisely what is needed in the marijuana agriculture sector. Since the marijuana industry has been operating in the shadows for decades, marijuana farmers are quite capable of evading onerous regulations. At least during the transition to legalization, it will be important for states to engage the marijuana farming community, and tailor regulations to obtain broad-based support for regulatory programs.

Nonetheless, developing effective water quality control programs for the marijuana industry will be challenging. First, given the federal marijuana prohibition, it is not clear that states will be empowered to use resources or programs fostered by the CWA. Although it would be difficult to distinguish marijuana-based agricultural runoff from general agricultural runoff, the federal government may not be supportive of programs that target and legitimize marijuana agriculture.

The 2010 Mendocino County, California, program mentioned earlier in this chapter was successful in partnering private growers with county officials to monitor plants and facilitate regulatory compliance, but a federal subpoena of the program's paperwork shut it down and broke up the partnership.[53] Many pollution control programs receive funding from the federal government and thus would be difficult to apply to marijuana farms without stoking fears of federal intervention.

In addition, because marijuana regulation is so novel, water pollution control programs will need to be coordinated with other governments and regulatory agencies. In May 2015, one month before Operation Emerald Tri-County conducted the raid on marijuana farms described earlier in this chapter, California's North Coast Regional Water Quality Control Board held a workshop in the area to discuss the board's proposed water quality regulations for marijuana cultivation.[54] The goal was to solicit input from marijuana farmers and invite them to participate in a mutually beneficial regulatory scheme. Farmers would be asked to clean up their operations and invest in water quality technologies, and in exchange, the board would give farmers cover to address water quality issues openly and legally.[55]

The workshop ended on a promising note,[56] but several weeks later, local sheriff's departments and the California Department of Fish and Wildlife conducted the Island Mountain raids, targeting farmers allegedly violating environmental regulations. The incident showed that without a clear framework for regulating marijuana farming, aspects of marijuana regulation like water quality control will suffer from a lack of coordination.

Outdoor marijuana farms may have adverse consequences for the environment, but indoor farms are not benign, either. The energy demands and carbon footprint of indoor grows have received widespread attention in both the press and academic scholarship.[57] Growing marijuana indoors requires high-intensity lighting, ventilation, and climate control systems, all of which are energy-intensive. A 2012 study found that the energy consumed by indoor marijuana farms alone constituted 1 percent of total electricity use in the United States, with carbon emissions reaching 15 million metric tons.[58] In California, indoor grows accounted for 3 percent of the state's total electricity use.[59]

Those estimates are likely obsolete now that more and more states are legalizing indoor marijuana cultivation.[60] In Colorado, for example, indoor marijuana farms comprise over half of new demand for power.[61] Power providers and state regulators are scrambling to adjust to rapid changes in the energy sector caused by these new and unprecedented demands.[62]

Unsurprisingly, the federal marijuana prohibition complicates energy regulation as well. Many utilities receive power from federal energy projects or facilities, are regulated directly or indirectly by federal agencies, or receive federal funding.[63] Accordingly, it is unclear if those utilities are legally permitted to provide energy for purposes of marijuana cultivation. The uncertainty has prompted some agencies to refrain from creating proactive regulations to address energy use by the marijuana industry.[64]

Some states have started to address the energy footprint of indoor grows. Approaches include a mix of sticks and carrots. In Oregon, where marijuana-induced energy demand led to several power outages in 2016, a trust provides cash incentives and technical assistance for cultivation operations.[65] Utilities in Denver, Colorado, and Seattle, Washington, similarly provide incentives in the form of efficient lighting upgrades or rebate programs.[66]

Marijuana licensing provides a fruitful opportunity to impose efficiency standards or clean energy requirements on marijuana farmers. Boulder, Colorado, and Humboldt County, California, for example, require indoor farming operations to obtain 100 percent of their energy needs from renewable energy sources.[67] In cases where renewable energy is not available to meet the demands of indoor operations, Boulder County imposes a tax on consumers (2.17 cents per kWh), the revenue from which funds sustainable marijuana cultivation projects and education programs.[68]

Another promising approach is to encourage or require indoor agricultural operations to schedule their light cycles to coincide with periods of low demand for the electrical grid as a whole. Off-peak hours typically are at night, while peak hours occur during the hottest periods of the day. But to plants grown indoors, outdoor conditions are irrelevant, and since off-peak energy is typically less expensive, there is reason to believe farmers will be enthusiastic about programs that facilitate "smart-metering" of electricity.[69] Electricity providers have an interest in preventing power shortages and blow-outs, and methods to reduce consumption during peak hours are becoming more sophisticated.

Policies designed to minimize the energy impacts of indoor farms could, of course, encourage or mandate that marijuana agriculture transition to outdoor environments, where solar energy is free and abundant. In certain climates, outdoor cultivation would be challenging, if not impossible.[70] But several states or local governments already require marijuana plants be grown indoors. They shouldn't be surprised by the staggering energy costs created by that policy preference. Simply allowing farmers to cultivate outside would represent a step in the right direction for the energy grid and the environment.

Aside from the energy demands, indoor growing operations must also address the sustainability of their growing methods. It is challenging for farmers to grow marijuana indoors on a commercial scale without the help of chemical fertilizers and pesticides. At the same time, regulators are requiring that marijuana products be vigorously tested and approved for sale and consumption by the public. Will indoor farms be able to comply with stringent testing protocols while remaining profitable?

In Colorado, where marijuana agriculture is dominated by indoor farms, the use of pesticides on marijuana has raised contentious issues. State lawmakers have received pressure from marijuana industry lobbyists to back off the pesticide issue. Indoor growers, on their part, are frustrated by the state's ignorance about marijuana cultivation. This disconnect has fostered little progress. One of the directors of the Colorado Department of Agriculture admitted that "the CDA has not actively sought to inspect and enforce the provisions of the [Colorado] Pesticide Applicator's Act on marijuana producers."[71]

Meanwhile, Colorado's marijuana consumers are losing confidence that their marijuana products are free from toxic or unhealthy levels of pesticides. Random tests have revealed the presence of several potent and unapproved pesticides in marijuana sold in licensed dispensaries. The city of Denver appears unwilling to wait for the state to make up its mind on this issue; its environmental health department confiscated 100,000 plants in 2015 to investigate potential pesticide violations.[72] Critics have accused the state of Colorado of bowing to the marijuana industry by not creating and enforcing a pesticide control program. Because consumers are preoccupied with the chemicals in their marijuana, some farmers have started marketing their marijuana as organically grown, even though that couldn't be further from the truth.

There is a robust market for organic agricultural products: in 2014, organic sales reached an estimated $39 billion, with a majority of Americans buying organic food.[73] The rationale is straightforward: as public awareness of the negative environmental and human health impacts associated with syn-thetic or nonorganic foods or food inputs grows, so too will the demand for alternative organic agricultural products.

One early impetus for this public awareness was Rachel Carson's *Silent Spring*, published in 1962, which identified pesticides such as DDT as the cause of a variety of observed ecological problems.[74] The book, along with growing public awareness and media coverage of environmental degrada-tion nationwide, prompted a broad response that included the passage of major state and federal environmental laws.[75] This recognition that human activities and natural systems were interconnected also prompted a return to organic farming,[76] and eventually, development of a federal organic cer-tification system.[77] The 1990 Organic Foods Production Act vested author-ity in the U.S. Department of Agriculture to develop organic certification regulations.[78] The National Organic Program is now the regulatory frame-work for organic agriculture and organic certification.[79]

It is not surprising, then, that there is also a market for organic mari-juana.[80] As public awareness of the environmental impacts of marijuana agriculture grows, so too does the pressure on marijuana farmers to adopt sustainable farming practices. The demand for organic marijuana has prompted a market response that parallels the market's response to organic foods in the 1970s. During that decade, in the absence of a federal regulatory framework, third-party organizations were created to provide independent certifications of organic agriculture. The Rodale Press established voluntary standards and a certification program, and helped organize the California Certified Organic Farmers and Oregon-Washington Tilth Organic Produc-ers Association.[81] States passed their own organic agriculture laws.[82] Oregon created the first state organic certification program, and by 1990, twenty-two states had developed some form of organic regulation.[83]

As the demand for organic products increased, however, these piecemeal approaches became problematic. Fraudulently labeled products flooded the market, state laws were inconsistent, and enforcement was unreliable.[84] The federal government stepped in to occupy the field of organic agriculture. The term "organic" has effectively been federalized, as agricultural products can be labeled organic only if they were grown in accordance with federal standards.[85] In addition, the federal government occupies the certification process, as the need for uniform federal certification standards and processes was a primary justification for federal organic legislation in the first place.[86]

In practice, enforcement of federal organic legislation often takes place at the state level by state officials promulgating organic certification programs, but these programs must be approved by the USDA and be in accordance with federal standards.[87] Thus, there is room for state involvement in the form of cooperative federalism,[88] but organic agriculture remains a federal field of regulation.

Because marijuana remains a controlled substance prohibited under federal law, and organic certification is a federal field of regulation, marijuana products cannot legally be labeled organic regardless of the method of cultivation.[89] As a consequence, the marijuana industry has established third-party certification programs that attempt to recognize organic marijuana agriculture in indirect ways. The certification programs mirror the USDA's organic agriculture requirements, but instead of using the "organic" label, programs use terms such as "naturally grown," "Clean Green certified," or "Certified Kind."[90] These programs compete with each other to represent the gold standard for organic agriculture, but as third-party certifiers their impact on the industry remains limited without a broader framework to evenly apply and enforce labeling standards. There is evidence that some marijuana being labeled and sold as "naturally grown" has not undergone certification of any kind.[91]

In Colorado, the Colorado Department of Agriculture provides organic certification and enforcement on behalf of the USDA.[92] Those obligations notwithstanding, the term "organic" has been used by many marijuana businesses in Colorado in their advertising, product labeling, and branding, with little to no state enforcement.[93]

Because the federal government occupies the field of organic certification, it will be difficult for states to develop their own organic marijuana programs. Amendments to state organic certification programs that incorporate marijuana agriculture are unlikely to be approved by the USDA. Absent robust certification frameworks, farmers will have few incentives to cultivate marijuana without synthetic pesticides or other substances that have adverse consequences for the environment and human health. At the same time, there will continue to be a market benefit conferred on businesses claiming to grow marijuana organically or naturally (regardless of the truth of those claims), and without an enforcement mechanism of some kind, consumers are likely to be misled or the terms will begin to lose meaning.

States and local governments can indirectly encourage organic marijuana cultivation by incorporating organic standards into their state or local cultivation licensing schemes. If these standards are enforced and well-communicated, farmers in that jurisdiction may be rewarded by higher prices.[94] More than likely, however, the organic marijuana industry will struggle to recognize and incentivize organic farming as long as the federal marijuana prohibition is maintained.

One of the most important influences on crop production is one that cannot be controlled: weather. Farmers can control or influence many aspects of cultivation, including soil conditions, crop type, and the timing of key activities like seed planting and crop harvesting, but the weather can be difficult to predict. Routine weather events that fluctuate mildly from expectations—more or less rain than anticipated, for example—can have significant consequences for crop yields.[95] But extreme weather events like droughts, freezes, floods, or fires can devastate crops, farmers, and, in turn, the stability of the market for an agricultural product.[96] In the face of climate change and an increase in weather uncertainty, developing resilience to environmental variability and extreme events will become an important goal of agricultural policy.[97]

If farmers were left to shoulder the burden of climatic uncertainty alone, rural economies and the country as a whole would likely suffer adverse consequences. Major crop failures could lead to farm failures, job losses, agribusiness failures, financial sector stress, and price increases. Farming would become more risky and less attractive. Recognizing this, U.S. agricultural policy has focused on two mechanisms to help farmers and the agricultural industry to develop resilience when dealing with uncertainty and crop failures.

The first mechanism consists of disaster relief. From 1989 to 2012, Congress made forty-two emergency funding appropriations that provided disaster relief to farmers in the amount of $70 billion.[98] Most of that total went directly to farmers to compensate for low commodity prices or crop failures.[99] Disaster relief can be an effective means of providing resilience and helping communities bounce back from disasters. Providing relief in the wake of natural disasters receives broad political support as well.[100]

But there are several problems with ad hoc disaster relief. First, the knowledge that governments will provide disaster funding may dissuade farmers from becoming more resilient, and they may fail to adjust their practices or not purchase crop insurance, for example.[101] This, in turn, makes farmers more dependent on disaster relief. Second, governments can't anticipate when disaster funding will be needed, creating a strain on budgets and financial planning.[102] These challenges combine to make ad hoc disaster funding unappealing in many contexts, including the agriculture industry, and have prompted Congress to pursue a second resilience mechanism: crop insurance. In 1938, Congress established the Federal Crop Insurance Program to support and regulate crop insurance.[103] Subsequent legislation has been enacted with the goal of making such insurance the primary risk management tool for the agriculture industry.[104]

Today the Federal Crop Insurance Corporation (FCIC) identifies eligible crops, sets premium rates, subsidizes premiums, and insures insurers.[105] As of 2014, 1.2 million crop insurance policies cover 130 crops, 294 million acres, and $110 billion in loss coverage.[106] Because the government subsidizes premiums (62 percent, on average) and covers administrative expenses,[107] the crop insurance program is one of the most costly components of federal agricultural policy.[108] Nonetheless, crop insurance and disaster relief payments create a major safety net for the agricultural industry.

Marijuana is not a crop eligible for crop insurance under the FCIC,[109] nor have marijuana farmers received federal disaster relief. This is to be expected, given the federal marijuana prohibition established by the Controlled Substances Act. But the federal prohibition has suppressed the emergence of marijuana crop insurance in the private sector as well, where most insurers are hesitant to become involved in an industry that remains illegal on the federal level.[110]

Without insurance or disaster relief, marijuana farmers are thus more vulnerable than other farmers to extreme events such as droughts, floods, and, increasingly, wildfires. California's drought history is well-chronicled,[111] and wildfires are particularly threatening to marijuana crops in the American West, many of which are grown in the wildland-urban interface where fires are most prevalent.[112] Floods and fires can wipe out crops altogether, while droughts and smoke can damage crop quality. Catastrophic crop losses can lead to the same consequences (farm failures, job losses, business failures, and price increases) for marijuana just as easily as for any other crop. Yet so far, states and private insurers have only tepidly explored the possibility of providing crop insurance to marijuana cultivators. Insurance for dispensaries has led the way, but crop insurance remains an undeveloped market tool.[113]

Courts have provided mixed support for marijuana farmers with these nascent insurance policies. In *Tracy v. USAA Casualty Ins.*, a federal court in Hawaii in 2012 agreed with an insurer that loss of state-legal marijuana plants was not a compensable claim under the insurance policy.[114] While the court found that state-legal marijuana plants are an insurable interest,[115] the federal marijuana prohibition preempts state marijuana law and makes the insurance policy (which purportedly covered the marijuana plants) an unenforceable contract contrary to public policy.[116]

In 2016, however, a federal court in Colorado pushed back on that view in *Green Earth Wellness Center LLC v. Atain Specialty Insurance Co.*, upholding the validity of an insurance policy's coverage of loss to marijuana plants and products from wildfire smoke damage.[117] Living plants were excluded from the policy in this instance, but the court rejected the idea that covered losses are not compensable because the federal prohibition makes insurance claims on marijuana a violation of federal law and public policy. "In light of several additional years evidencing a continued erosion of any clear and consistent federal public policy in this area," the court declined to follow *Tracy*, instead finding valid contractual claims in which both parties intended to cover marijuana products as insurable commodities.[118]

The *Tracy* and *Green Earth* decisions are in conflict with each other, and it remains to be seen how other courts will address the validity of insurance policies covering marijuana, and in particular marijuana crops. The *Green Earth* decision paves the way for marijuana farmers to obtain and enforce private crop insurance, though courts might be more willing to find preemption concerns because crop insurance is extensively regulated on the federal level.

In any case, without agricultural support programs like disaster relief or crop insurance, marijuana farmers and marijuana farming communities will remain vulnerable to extreme events. This lack of support may also dissuade existing farmers of insured crops from incorporating marijuana into their crop portfolios, thus suppressing the normalization of marijuana cultivation. Intrepid private insurers may be able to provide some relief in response to market demands, but the validity of marijuana insurance, and marijuana crop insurance, remains unsettled as a matter of law. As a consequence, the marijuana industry will not have at its disposal a primary tool for agricultural risk management for the foreseeable future.

There is a future in which marijuana agriculture is appropriately regulated and farmers are aware of their environmental responsibilities. The ecological impacts are minimized, while farmers who employ the most sustainable farming methods are rewarded for their efforts. The marijuana industry isn't there yet, obviously. But it should be encouraging that many marijuana farming communities are actively involved in crafting environmental regulations for their industry, aware that they're under pressure to create a sustainable product.

It may also be helpful that the marijuana industry is still characterized by hundreds of thousands of relatively small-scale indoor and outdoor growing operations. While the fragmentation of the agricultural community might make it harder for regulators to monitor the landscape, hopefully this fragmentation will prevent regulators from being unduly influenced by oligopolies and their lobbyists. In addition, the farming community may be able to avert some of the large-scale environmental impacts created by industrial monoculture operations in the past.

Perhaps I am being too optimistic about the sustainability of small-scale farming, though. Jonathan Caulkins of Carnegie Mellon University dismissed my suggestion that environmental impacts will be a major challenge for the marijuana industry in the future. "Environmental issues are probably really quite unimportant," he argued. If one large-scale farm can capture the market, he said, the environmental impacts will be concentrated and minimal in the long run. "Even if the 10,000 acres are not farmed in a sustainable way, that's a round-off error compared to all of American agriculture. In that sense the environmental side doesn't matter much at the national level."

I've argued throughout this book that marijuana farmers and the public would not benefit from a Big Marijuana takeover that concentrates farming in a handful of large-scale farms. Family farmers would be out of jobs, rural economies would suffer, the craft and connoisseur markets would regress, and consumer choices would dwindle. There is at least one other downside as well: the environmental public health implications of dirt-cheap marijuana.

Because many drug and alcohol users have substance abuse problems, the public has an interest in preventing the price of an intoxicant from collapsing. Artificially high prices may not keep an intoxicant out of the hands of a substance abuser completely, but they do impose some limits on consumption. A price floor can be maintained by imposing taxes, of course. Or it can be maintained by forcing the industry to adopt inefficient modes of production.

The idea that a marijuana price collapse could create a public health concern represents another opportunity for small-scale marijuana farmers. Keeping the farming community fragmented into hundreds of thousands of relatively small farms is, technically, inefficient. Spending years creating new, interesting strains is, technically, inefficient. Protecting designations of origin is, technically, inefficient. And if one sprawling Big Marijuana farm could supply the national market for marijuana, then maybe worrying about all these environmental impacts is, technically, inefficient too.

But marijuana farmers are in a unique position to argue that these inefficiencies are an asset, not a liability. Not only do all these inefficiencies yield a higher-quality, more sustainable product, but they also keep prices from collapsing, which would exacerbate public health problems. I am not terribly concerned that a marijuana price collapse is a public health disaster waiting to happen.[119] But many Americans are anxious about the effects marijuana legalization will have on society. The family farming model—and its attendant inefficiencies—may provide an opportunity for sustainable agriculture and public health advocates to converge.

Is family farming the most efficient mode of production? No, probably not. But it is in the public interest.

9 Big Hemp, Small Weed

Hemp ... is abundantly productive and will grow forever on the same spot.
—Thomas Jefferson, third president of the United States[1]

The 115th United States Congress will not be remembered for its bipartisan bridge-building. Partisan festivities kicked off in January 2017, as the Republican-controlled Congress condemned President Obama's decision to adopt new regulations during his last days in command of the federal government. Once the Trump administration was in office, many of these regulations were promptly rolled back. Most of 2017 was spent trying to repeal the Affordable Care Act—perhaps the Obama administration's signature domestic achievement—despite the resistance of congressional Democrats.

The highlight (or low point, depending on your political views) of the 115th Congress's first year in office represented a brazenly partisan triumph. After months of successfully refusing to hold hearings on President Obama's nominee for a Supreme Court vacancy, Senate Republicans made history by invoking the "nuclear option" to end debate on President Trump's nominee for the vacancy, clearing the way for the Senate's confirmation. The whole campaign was an unprecedented masterstroke of partisan politicking.[2]

The brains behind the operation was Senate Majority Leader Mitch McConnell, a Republican from Kentucky. Suffice it to say there is no love lost between McConnell and congressional Democrats. In an attempt to block President Trump's Supreme Court nominee, Senator Jeff Merkley of Oregon spent over fifteen hours on the Senate floor, the eighth-longest floor speech since 1900.[3] At some point during that fifteen hours, Merkley accused Senate Republicans of "stealing" the Supreme Court seat, calling McConnell's campaign a "warfare tactic of partisanship."[4] McConnell wasn't fazed; he invoked the nuclear option the next day, ending debate.

This wasn't the first time McConnell and Merkley faced off. As the chief deputy whip for Senate Democrats, Merkley is responsible for ensuring that his party colleagues line up against McConnell's legislative proposals. McConnell, the leader of his party in the Senate, is a staunch Republican, while Merkley is a progressive Democrat, the only Senator to endorse liberal firebrand Bernie Sanders in the 2016 Democratic presidential primaries. The two have opposite views on issues ranging from banking reform to environmental protection.

You'd be forgiven for thinking McConnell and Merkley would have no use for each other. But that is not the case. There is one issue that unites them: American hemp. In June 2017, just two months after McConnell and Merkley went head to head on the Supreme Court vacancy, the two co-sponsored a Senate resolution designating the week of June 5–11 as "Hemp History Week."

The resolution—which received unanimous support from the Senate—explains that the goals of Hemp History Week are to "commemorate the historical relevance of industrial hemp in the United States and to promote the full growth potential of the industrial hemp industry."[5] While the resolution is mostly symbolic, McConnell, Merkley, and their state colleagues in the Senate (Kentucky's Rand Paul and Oregon's Ron Wyden) have introduced legislation that would lift federal restrictions on hemp cultivation. They appear determined to stay at it until they succeed.[6]

How can politicians from opposite ends of the ideological spectrum set aside their differences for the sake of legalizing hemp farming, even at a time of such bitter partisanship? Part of the answer is local. Kentucky has at various times been the country's largest producer of industrial hemp, and the state's farmers are eager to reclaim the throne.[7] Oregon farmers, meanwhile, have embraced the potential of hemp after the state legalized cannabis cultivation in 2014.[8]

But the senators from Kentucky and Oregon also realize that the federal prohibition on hemp farming has national and international implications as well. As they stated in their resolution: "the United States is the largest consumer of hemp products in the world, but the United States is the only major industrialized country that restricts hemp farming."[9] The U.S. market for hemp products has been estimated at nearly $600 million. But without a domestic farming industry to produce the hemp going into those products, the U.S. market must rely on imports (China is the largest hemp fiber supplier to the United States, while Canada is the largest hemp seed supplier).[10] There is no agricultural reason American farmers couldn't fulfill these demands for hemp instead. Farmers were cultivating hemp in the United States on a large scale as recently as World War II, after all.

Loosening restrictions on hemp farming appears to have both bipartisan support and national appeal. The 2013 Farm Bill signed into law by President Obama included a provision (known as the "McConnell Hemp Provision") that authorized universities and state agencies to launch hemp farming pilot programs in states where hemp cultivation is legal. Many states are taking advantage—there are now at least thirty states that have loosened restrictions on hemp farming or authorized it altogether. The Industrial Hemp Farming Act,[11] which would exclude industrial hemp from the Controlled Substances Act's definition of marijuana, increasingly enjoys bipartisan support.[12]

Hemp still has some detractors, however. The U.S. Drug Enforcement Administration (DEA), most prominently, has expressed concern that law enforcement will have a hard time distinguishing between hemp farms and marijuana farms; they fear this confusion could provide cover for marijuana farmers to engage in illicit cultivation. Farmers still need a permit from the DEA to cultivate hemp, and the permit application process is often long and arduous; as a result, some states and hemp farmers are starting to ignore the federal application process. The DEA has also intervened when farmers try to import viable seeds for cultivation, seizing hundreds of pounds of hemp seeds from Kentucky farmers in 2014. Still, the DEA's position is not anti-hemp so much as it is anti-marijuana, as the agency's resistance to hemp farming appears to result from the plant's association with its psychoactive relative.[13]

It may not be long until hemp farming is legal at both state and federal levels in the United States. But the paths to legalizing hemp look quite different at the two levels. The federal legalization movement is proceeding in spite of its relation to marijuana—the strategy so far is to distinguish hemp and marijuana from one another. But at the state level, the legalization of hemp farming is occurring because of its relation to marijuana—in many cases, hemp farming is legal because it is now legal to farm cannabis in general. This difference has interesting implications for the cannabis industry, including both hemp and marijuana farmers. Since hemp has two paths toward legalization (general cannabis legalization and specific hemp legalization), it may become a completely legal crop before marijuana does. This, in turn, might force the hemp farming community and the marijuana farming community (and the laws governing both) to go their separate ways.

That would be unfortunate, in my view. Hemp and marijuana have their differences, and those differences are reflected in the way the two crops are farmed. But hemp and marijuana are both strains of cannabis, and their genetic similarities are close enough that hemp and marijuana farmers would benefit from working together to create a cannabis agriculture industry that is sustainable and productive. This book has largely focused on the future of marijuana farming. But that future isn't complete if American hemp farming isn't a part of it.

Extolling the virtues of hemp is a time-honored tradition. Ancient China's "God Farmer"—Emperor Shennong—may have been one of the first to do so around 4,500 years ago, and his praise has since been echoed by prominent historical figures such as Confucius and Queen Elizabeth I.[14] Senators McConnell and Merkley are the latest in a long line of American hemp proponents that includes George Washington, John Adams, and Thomas Jefferson. When Jack Herer wrote *The Emperor Wears No Clothes* (also known as the "Hemp Bible"), he awakened in readers and advocates a passion for hemp that the prohibition era had sought to suppress.[15] The case for hemp was too compelling to ignore.

Even in ancient times hemp was a versatile crop. It could be used for fiber to make rope or textiles, or the seeds could be used for food or oil. Today the versatility has magnified. Hemp is used in an estimated 25,000 products worldwide, including applications for agriculture, textiles, recycling, transportation, furniture, food and beverages, paper, construction materials, and personal care.[16] Hemp can be grown to produce biomass and converted into energy, or it can be grown to produce food for humans or livestock. Hemp fiber can be used to produce a beautiful archival hemp canvas, and hempseed oil can be used to produce the paint brushed onto the canvas. The possibilities, as far as we know today, are endless.

From a farmer's point of view, hemp has its costs and benefits. The main challenge when growing hemp is accessing its valuable internal fibers, which are protected by a hard outer-tissue layer called the hurd. For thousands of years, hemp farmers have broken down the hurd by cutting the plants down and letting them lie in a field for a few weeks. During that time, natural elements like sun, rain, and fungus cause the hurd to decompose and provide access to the internal fibers.[17] This is a rudimentary and labor-intensive process, but, remarkably, most modern hemp farmers still rely on this harvesting method, and hemp farming remains profitable nonetheless. As the industry develops, technological innovations will most likely enable farmers to access the internal fibers without needing to wait for nature to break down the hurd. Some inventions claiming to do just that are already on the market.[18]

The second challenge for American hemp farmers is that "hemp," like "marijuana," is another catchall term for a category of plants that contains many different strains. Some strains have been developed to favor yields of one of the plant's three usable parts (the seed, fiber, and hurd) over the others, for example. And like marijuana strains, some hemp strains are better suited to certain environments. The challenge for American hemp farmers is to figure out which of the many hemp strains in existence will grow well on their farm. The experimental pilot programs authorized by the 2013 Farm Bill should offer some insights, and other governments (Canada and the United Kingdom, for example) publish databases that provide guidance to hemp farmers. But some experimentation will still be necessary—American hemp farmers don't have the head start marijuana farmers enjoy thanks to their marijuana-breeding predecessors.

Despite the challenges, the benefits of farming hemp are considerable. All three of the plant's usable parts can be harvested and sold commercially, thus increasing the plant's profitability. For example, the fibers could be sold to a construction materials manufacturer, the hurd could be sold to a biomass combustion company, and the seed could be sold to an oil processor (or, with a moderate investment, processed into oil right on the farm).[19] For a farmer, these options provide resilience and flexibility. If the market for one of the parts dries up for a while, the other two markets can minimize the losses. By keeping a foot in each of these doors, a farmer keeps sight of what is going on inside.

Hemp can also be used rotationally in order to reclaim or maintain soil quality for other crops. Hemp seeds put down long root systems in a matter of weeks, breaking up overworked, compacted, or arid soils. The American hemp farmers of the past would often plant hemp to ready a field for another crop, or rotate hemp in with other crops on a seasonal basis.[20] Anything that can be harvested and sold from these hemp plants is a bonus, while the organic matter left behind after the harvest composts to create nutrient rich soil for the next planting season.

The challenging harvesting process notwithstanding, hemp is a fairly low-maintenance crop to grow. Strains have been adapted to grow in virtually any agricultural region on earth. Little to no pesticides (including herbicides, fungicides, or rodenticides) are needed for the plant to grow vigorously. It also requires less water compared to other crops used to produce fibers, oils, or biomass. Not only do these factors make hemp plants relatively easy to grow, they also reduce the environmental impact of hemp farming and lower production costs for farmers.

Zooming out from this farm-level perspective, the big-picture benefits should be readily apparent. Monoculture crops are known to be reducing soil quality across the United States. Pesticides and other additives are difficult to regulate and may be harmful to human health and wildlife. Agriculture is already the largest water user in the country and the world. Hemp farming alleviates all of these concerns, requiring less water and pesticides than many other crops. On top of all this, hemp farming is the starting point for a billion-dollar industry with an endless list of product manufacturers waiting to get their hands on some hemp, a plant oozing with potential.

Unsurprisingly, perhaps, the hemp farming community is facing many of the same questions facing the marijuana farming community, which I've explored in this book.

The first question, inevitably, is whether hemp farming will be profitable when legalization invites an influx of farmers to start cultivating and selling hemp. Canadian hemp farmers appear to be doing quite well—many are making millions of dollars in profits annually.[21] But they are taking advantage of the U.S. prohibition on hemp farming by tapping into the American hemp market, with little outside competition. Will the market stay profitable once American farmers get in the game too?

A report commissioned by the Congressional Research Service surveyed market studies on the growth potential of the hemp farming industry. Many studies show a generally positive outlook, citing the growing list of products that use hemp, the low maintenance requirements of the crop, the soil reclamation or rotation crop potential, and a rise in consumer demand.[22]

Other studies are more skeptical, and point to widespread uncertainties inherent in an emerging market as reason for caution.

Government policies play a part in this equation as well. Burdensome licensing processes, excessive fees, or crushing taxes can doom a hemp farm before it ever gets off the ground. Subsidies, by contrast, grease the wheels of production. The European Union subsidizes hemp farming to the tune of four hundred dollars per acre in order to encourage production.[23]

A corollary to the profitability question is the level to which the hemp farming community will consolidate. Will hemp farming become the vocation of small or medium-scale family farms, or will it consolidate into a few large-scale operations?

Unlike marijuana, which is a high-maintenance plant and is typically inhaled or ingested by consumers, hemp is a low-maintenance plant that becomes an industrial input to other products. There is less of a craft or local consumer preference for products like biomass fuel, paper, or insulation materials. Also, the hemp harvesting process is so demanding that it's possible its cultivation will be profitable only on a large scale. One Canadian hemp company thought the minimum acreage necessary to cultivate hemp profitably might be 1,000 to 3,000 acres.[24] Hemp may, therefore, be well suited for commoditization.

As the current global market for industrial hemp suggests, it is in fact already an agricultural commodity. The European Union subsidizes hemp farming partly because hemp shows promise as a versatile and sustainable commodity, and partly so that the E.U.'s hemp farmers can compete in the global marketplace for a product that lacks unique qualities.

If hemp is merely an industrial input, its craft or artisanal potential is limited. But hemp isn't limited to industrial applications. One of the largest hemp markets is in hempseed oil and the hempseed cake left over after the oil is processed. Both products can be used in foods and beverages, and are increasingly trendy items in grocery stores or farmer's markets. It's not hard to envision someone who's already making a kale-banana-almond milk smoothie adding hempseed oil for a dash of healthy protein. In fact, when I Googled "most hipster smoothie" to get some ideas on ingredients to throw into the previous sentence, the first recipe that came up called for hempseeds. "I love hemp seeds," the author of the recipe admitted.[25] Next, consumers might be loving organic, locally grown, family-farm-supporting hempseeds.

Another reason to doubt the total consolidation of hemp farming is the fact that hemp might be cultivated by thousands of existing family farmers. The marijuana industry is already dominated by tens of thousands (if not hundreds of thousands) of small-scale farms, and they won't go down without a fight. The American hemp industry is not similarly characterized, since the crop has been largely forgotten for several decades.

But hemp is a more natural fit alongside other existing crops on family farms. Because marijuana is a high-maintenance plant, with peculiar needs and a high level of expertise needed to cultivate it to perfection, it makes sense that marijuana farmers tend to be specialists. Hemp could be more easily incorporated into a farmer's existing crop portfolio, though, either by rotating it in with their other crops to work the soil or by gradually refining their cultivating methods. As one hemp farmer put it, "farming is farming."[26] If the adoption rate is high enough, states will have an interest in protecting their cottage industries, and may take steps to prevent agribusiness giants from taking over the market.

Finally, like the marijuana industry, the hemp industry will need to reckon with the complex genetics of the cannabis plant. The remarkable ability of the cannabis genus to breed and create new plants capable of adapting to virtually any agricultural environment is a testament to the genus's resilience. Its versatility also provides the farming community with a wealth of options to experiment with. Might it also create a race to patent hemp strains or trademark hemp brands?

In the United States, hemp strains are just as eligible to receive patents as marijuana strains are. In fact, the bulk of the cannabis strains that have been issued patents by the U.S. Patent and Trademark Office are for nonpsychoactive cannabis strains, or hemp. Not much is known about which hemp strains will grow most vigorously in this country, but if a few patent holders end up owning the intellectual property rights to the few strains that grow well in the arid American West, or the humid Southeast, they could effectively corner the market.

It is unclear whether governments or consumers will be enthusiastic about genetically modified hemp, either. The Canadian government preemptively banned hemp GMOs before they hit the market. South of the border, however, the climate for GMOs is friendlier. When North Dakota legalized hemp cultivation, it touted the fact that University of North Dakota researchers were working on a genetic modification that would make hemp easier to distinguish from marijuana.[27] Since hemp is an industrial input to many products, perhaps the market will invite the development of hemp GMOs.

Hemp farming is also much more likely than marijuana farming to scale up and produce a generic commodity. Hemp fibers and biomass products are, for the most part, fairly indistinct from one another, and they aren't directly consumed by people. The harvesting process is still so laborious that a hemp farm might need to be hundreds or thousands of acres in size in order to benefit from economies of scale. Nevertheless, there are reasons to believe hemp will have a role to play on the American family farm, since it is a useful rotation crop and soil remediator, and it might not be very hard for an experienced farmer to grow. Finally, there is the possibility that hempseed oil might even have a terroir. If so, perhaps hemp might develop a craft market after all.

If hempseed products reveal the terroir of the farm they were cultivated on, that might provide a justification for hemp appellations. Even if that's not the case (and admittedly, it may seem like a stretch), incorporating hemp farming into the same organizational model as marijuana farming wouldn't be a bad idea. The two communities need to work out some kind of arrangement, for the simple reason that hemp and marijuana should not be grown in close proximity to one another.

Unlike most plants, cannabis is a dioecious species, meaning the individual plants can be male or female.[28] Marijuana crops are grown using exclusively female cannabis plants. This limits the presence of unwanted seeds, while simultaneously increasing yields of THC-producing buds.[29] Unfortunately for marijuana farmers, cannabis plants can be pollinated across large distances.[30] Even if one farmer eradicates all the male plants on her farm, a slightly less scrupulous farmer next door who lets a male plant mature to reproduction could accidentally pollinate not only his female plants, but all the female plants in his neighborhood as well. When female plants are pollinated, their flowers produce seeds and stop growing as vigorously, reducing the quality and yield of marijuana crops.

Strains of industrial hemp are not exclusively female, but cross-pollination is equally undesirable. Across the United States, wherever states have permitted the cultivation of industrial hemp, its classification as such is at least partly determined by THC content.[31] The federal 2013 Farm Bill, as well, defines hemp as "the plant Cannabis sativa L. and any part of such plant, whether growing or not, with a delta-9 tetrahydrocannabinol concentration of not more than 0.3 percent on a dry weight basis."[32]

If marijuana strains pollinate a hemp crop, the THC content of the plants is likely to increase above legal limits.[33] That would make the crop unmarketable for hemp applications, and since the hemp farmer likely would not have a marijuana cultivation license, he or she could not sell the crop as psychoactive marijuana, either. Even if the farmer did hold a license—or, more likely, tried to sell the tainted crop on the black market—the hemp/marijuana hybrid product would probably be so unusual and low-quality from a marijuana consumer's perspective that it would be unmarketable. Economic considerations aside, if a hemp farmer inadvertently produces psychoactive marijuana in a state where marijuana cultivation remains illegal, the farmer could be at risk of criminal or civil penalties. It is desirable, therefore, to maintain a healthy distance between regions cultivating marijuana and regions cultivating hemp. Logically, navigating this botanical idiosyncrasy will require cooperation within the cannabis agriculture community.

A laissez-faire approach that does not address the potential for cross-pollination would likely disrupt crop production. The threat of cross-pollination is not unique to cannabis; corn and beet farmers must also cooperate to avoid cross-pollination from wild or genetically variable crops.[34] Hemp and marijuana farmers can look to farmers of other crops, then, to find cooperation mechanisms that can ensure cross-pollination is prevented or minimized.

There are several well-known agricultural techniques that farmers and agricultural regulators use to minimize cross-pollination or cross-fertilization, many of which require crops to be isolated in one fashion or another.[35] Spatial isolation can be achieved by creating isolation distance requirements that place crops a minimum distance from one another.[36] This approach would require intense monitoring, and given the distances cannabis pollen can travel, may be ineffectual or impracticable for hemp farming. Spatial isolation has nevertheless been a popular option for regulators. Canada has adopted distance requirements for hemp farms, with the distance required between farms dependent on the type of hemp being cultivated. Washington State's license rules for hemp farming require that industrial hemp "not be grown within four miles of any field or facility being used to grow marijuana."[37]

Alternatively, planting dates for hemp and marijuana crops could be staggered so that plants flower or mature at different intervals, thus achieving temporal isolation.[38] Staggering flowering times is challenging, however, when strains are diversified and weather conditions defy expectations. This approach also requires intense coordination between neighboring farmers, a potentially unrealistic expectation.

A third strategy would physically isolate crops by requiring them to be bagged or covered when mature. Applying this method to marijuana and hemp cultivation would effectively mandate indoor agriculture, a heavy-handed approach from a regulatory perspective and one with severe energy security implications.[39]

Marijuana farmers could take males out of the picture entirely if regulators or farming cooperatives allow the propagation of clones. Because clones of a female plant will always be female, a male plant doesn't need to be kept around for reproductive purposes. While marijuana genetics haven't developed to the point that cloning could stand on its own (some base of seeded plants is still necessary to resist senescence), the use of clones would help a region reduce the likelihood of cross-pollination.

Farmers could also agree to cultivate only one crop type (marijuana or hemp) in a given agricultural region. The climatic preferences of hemp and marijuana suggest this approach is preferable from an agricultural point of view. Marijuana has a smaller footprint and thrives in mountainous Mediterranean zones (with wet winters and hot, dry summers), whereas industrial hemp can be grown in wetter, colder climates,[40] and in vast, dense fields.[41]

Appellations represent a natural mechanism that could be used to facilitate cooperation between hemp and marijuana farmers. By establishing cultivation rules and standards for each region, appellations cater to the region's topographical and agricultural strengths. Appellations could be designated as marijuana-producing or hemp-producing, or they could facilitate the more involved cooperation required if crops are grown in close proximity to each other. The former approach may be more pragmatic; in Oregon, appellations are already being proposed for exactly this purpose.[42]

Courtney Moran has carved out a niche as an Oregon attorney and hemp farming advocate. In 2014, when the state legalized cannabis cultivation, she wondered why no one was applying for a license to grow hemp. Oregon farmers were sitting back and waiting, even though hemp cultivation was now legal under both state and federal law. So Moran worked with a farmer and wrote up a permit application on his behalf. The application was denied, but the process put her right in the middle of an exciting new industry.

She continued working with farmers and state regulators to develop a hemp farming industry in Oregon. By February of 2015, the first license was issued, and eleven farmers were licensed to grow hemp that summer.

It took only one summer for cross-pollination to occur. Hemp farms, to that point massively outnumbered by Oregon's marijuana farms, were pollinating marijuana crops, while marijuana crops were pollinating the hemp crops. In response, the larger marijuana industry lobbied the state to place a moratorium on hemp farming. At the end of that first summer, the state's Department of Agriculture issued a notice announcing that no further hemp cultivation licenses would be issued. It could have dealt a fatal blow to Oregon hemp farmers.

Moran and a passionate hemp farmer decided they couldn't let the industry die so soon. They created the Oregon Industrial Hemp Farmers Association, an organization that works closely with the Department of Agriculture to work out the kinks in existing rules and industry practices. The department welcomed the input, and put the industry back on track. By May 2017, 175 farmers were licensed to cultivate hemp in the state.

Moran favors a self-regulated approach to the cannabis industry's organizational issues. Farmers and regulators have so much yet to learn about hemp, marijuana, and cross-pollination that it might not make sense to create and enforce rules right away if those rules are merely stabs in the dark. "We encourage responsible family farming," she told me. That would appear to be the state's position as well. Oregon has not imposed distance requirements between hemp and marijuana plants, as some fear that could lead to litigation. For now, farmers on both sides seem to have reached an unsteady compromise.[43]

Regardless of the approach taken by states or the cannabis agriculture industry, the cultivation of industrial hemp and marijuana is likely to increase dramatically in the coming months and years as legal restrictions on farmers are relaxed. For many reasons—including the need to minimize cross-pollination between hemp and marijuana crops—it is essential that farmers and regulators coordinate this growth in agricultural development.

Appellations are a promising mechanism to minimize disruption between farmers and to ensure that cannabis agriculture grows smoothly and strategically. But other mechanisms might work just as well, if not better. There are early signs—in Oregon, for example—that cannabis farmers are not all on the same page. But for now they share at least one common bond: they exist precariously as family farms in an industry that is changing rapidly. To survive, cannabis farmers will need to put aside their differences and work together to create an industry rooted in the ideals of family farming.

It will take time to rebuild the American hemp farming industry. Since the federal government last encouraged farmers to cultivate hemp during World War II, the crop has gone dormant on U.S. soil. A verified seed stock tailored for U.S. climates doesn't exist anymore, and will need to be pieced together using strains developed in other countries. Over time, the ingenuity of American breeders and farmers will create strains adapted to each microregion in the country. But that moment is, for now, not imminent.

In the meantime, the hemp farming community will need to address many of the same questions being faced by the country's first legal marijuana farmers. Will farming be profitable? Can family farms survive? Can the two cannabis crops coexist?

Joy Beckerman, one of the nation's foremost hemp experts and hemp farming advocates, doesn't have all the answers, but she thinks we're on the right path to figuring them out. A self-described "hard-core hippie sister," Beckerman first learned about the benefits of industrial hemp from a flyer passed out at a Grateful Dead concert in 1990. As both a single mother and an only child raised by a single father, Beckerman developed a keen intolerance for injustice that drew her to push back on the cannabis prohibition in whatever way she could.

As a hemp farming advocate, Beckerman is torn when I ask her about Big Agriculture producers getting in on the hemp industry. "I'm going to put my hemp industry hat on, then I'm going to put my hippie girl hat on," she warns me. "I encourage industrial hemp production on a large scale and on a small scale. ... If Jolly Green Giant wants to plant 20,000 acres of hemp, I would be jumping up and down! But I trust we are evolving as a species, and realize Big Ag is not only not regenerative, but not sustainable. How can we feel good about introducing this ancient, incredible, valuable crop, if all it's going to be is another agricultural commodity to ruin the land with? We have to develop new regenerative agricultural techniques. What I'd like to see, whether we're talking hemp or strawberries, the answer is the same. We would rather encourage small, local, organic farms."

As for the cultural and horticultural differences between hemp and marijuana that are threatening to tear the cannabis industry apart, Beckerman agrees with Moran that the farming community and the market should be given the chance to figure things out on their own before the government gets involved. The answers to the industry's most pressing agricultural questions, after all, might be right in front of us, in the plant that raised all these questions in the first place.

"It's more about cannabis and the many, many lessons that it's teaching us," she said. "It's teaching us how to be good neighbors, and good farmers. It's teaching us how to live with each other."

The welfare of the farmer is vital to that of the whole country.
—William Howard Taft, twenty-seventh president of the United States[1]

The proper role of government ... is that of partner with the farmer—never his master. By every possible means we must develop and promote that partnership—to the end that agriculture may continue to be a sound, enduring foundation for our economy and that farm living may be a profitable and satisfying experience.
—Dwight D. Eisenhower, thirty-forth president of the United States[2]

One thousand years ago, tribal migrants settled into a fertile valley along the Trinity River in northern California. The valley is located near the Trinity's confluence with the Klamath River, providing human settlers with plentiful fish stocks and an abundance of edible plants and game animals. The migrants established themselves as the Hoopa tribe, and lived in relative isolation in the valley for hundreds of years.

In 1864, the Hoopas reluctantly signed a treaty with the U.S. government that set aside lands in the valley for the Hoopa Valley Indian Reservation. The treaty allowed the Hoopa to stay on their ancestral lands, one of a small handful of tribes that weren't forcibly removed from their homes. But the tribe's relationship with the federal government quickly soured. A decade after signing the treaty, federal officials contemplated relocating the Hoopa further south, to a reservation set aside to house a half-dozen disparate tribes being driven from their homelands. The Hoopa sent one of their most prominent members—a man named James Jackson—to negotiate a resolution with the government. Jackson was a farmer, judge, and tribal leader, and commanded the respect of federal officials. He won the right for the Hoopa to stay in the Hoopa Valley.[3]

Over the next several decades, the Hoopa developed a talent for agriculture. Historically reliant on aquaculture and traditional hunting and gathering techniques, the Hoopa were encouraged by the valley's favorable climate, plentiful water, and rich soils to turn to farming instead.[4] Hoopa farmers traded with neighboring tribes and white settlements, and adopted European agricultural methods. Much to the frustration of federal officials, however, the Hoopa's adoption of white practices was selective. The tribe embraced modern farming without losing their tribal identity, religious practices, or cultural traditions.[5]

Unfortunately, there weren't enough arable lands in the Hoopa Valley to go around. A federal agent observed that by the 1890s farming had possibly become too popular on the Hoopa Valley Reservation: "The success of a few who first adopted this work encouraged the others, so that at present time the question is not, how shall I induce others to cultivate land, but where shall I find land for them to cultivate."[6] At the time, federal officials were trying to determine how to divide the Hoopa Valley Reservation into plots they could allocate to individual Hoopa tribal members. The effort was part of a broader strategy designed to assimilate tribes into mainstream American culture. By transferring tribal lands to individual Native Americans, the government hoped they would either adopt European-American lifestyles or eventually sell their land to white settlers. On the surface, the allotments seemed generous. But in reality, they embodied a cynical deprivation of tribal resources.

The Hoopa, by several accounts, didn't fall for the trappings of the federal government's allotment strategy. They accepted the land transfers, but did not allow private ownership of tribal lands to erode their cultural identities or economic customs. Many of the allotments reflected preexisting arrangements between neighbors, and the scarcity of arable land forced Hoopa farmers to cultivate their crops on small-scale plots that encouraged subsistence farming.

Nonetheless, farming in the valley was dense and intense, and eventually soil quality and crop production diminished. James Jackson was concerned that white settlers would try to claim the Hoopa tribe's surrounding natural resources, and pushed federal officials to allot the tribe's undeveloped lands to its members so they could have more space to farm sustainably. The federal government was happy to comply, allotting timber and grazing acreage to Hoopa members in 1918. Jackson and other leaders did their best to make sure these allotments didn't break up the tribe. Jackson himself consented to the transfer of his landholdings, and offered his farming equipment whenever a group of Hoopa farmers were getting together to work the harvest.

Over time the allotment strategy succeeded in anglicizing some aspects of Hoopa culture, but for the most part, the tribe stuck together, refusing to be assimilated into mainstream American culture. Federal officials had a hard time making sense of it all. One observer captured the tribe's surprising cohesion:

> During the twenties, everybody had a little farm here and that's how they made their living. Everybody would help one another. They would say, "I'll help you next week and you can help me," and that's the way they got by. There was no money involved.[7]

The Hoopa couldn't insulate themselves from the unrelenting might of the federal government forever. But a steely resolve and commitment to one another kept the community alive and the tribe's values intact. As a tribal historian put it, "the people's quiet, persistent refusal to abandon ancient beliefs had itself become a way of life in Hoopa Valley."[8]

Nearly a hundred years later, I'm listening to James Jackson's great-grandson lay out his vision for the Hoopa tribe's resurgence. It's the hottest part of the day on a hot day in May, and Sonny Jackson and I are taking refuge in his trailer overlooking the Trinity River. Like his great-grandfather, Sonny is passionate about the well-being of his people, and today he's particularly fired up about it. We're talking about a proposal Sonny had put forward to the members of the Hoopa Valley Tribe about a year ago, a proposal the tribe ultimately rejected.

Sonny has a plan that he thinks will revitalize the tribe, creating jobs and income for tribal members, while generating enough collective wealth to fund educational and rehabilitation programs. The plan would require tribal members to form and maintain a farming cooperative. The farm would tap into the Hoopa tribe's historic agricultural strengths, while bringing the community together with a unified mission. The only problem? Sonny wants the farming cooperative to grow marijuana.

Sonny Jackson grew up in the Hoopa Valley Reservation. He served his country in Vietnam after high school, and when he came back home in 1970, the marijuana game had exploded. Good seeds were coming over from Asia, and northern California farmers were learning how to grow highgrade product. Sonny and his cousin Arthur became two of the most prolific marijuana farmers in the region in short order, in part because local law enforcement was hesitant to encroach onto tribal lands. But federal officials didn't share those concerns. For a while they coordinated with the Hoopa tribe to take down the valley's most notorious farmers. Sonny disliked the high-stakes militarized zone the area had become, so he left the reservation in 1980. He didn't come back for twenty years.

By the time he returned, marijuana farming had changed again. California's medical marijuana laws had loosened penalties and redirected law enforcement priorities. The feds weren't hitting tribal lands as hard anymore. Slowly but surely, Sonny and Arthur built their farming business back up again. By 2017, they were leasing farmlands across the valley and employing a modest workforce to cultivate elusive strains of high-quality outdoor marijuana. It's a demanding lifestyle, but they make a good living for themselves.

Perhaps because he's a Jackson—part of a prominent family known for providing leadership to the Hoopa community—Sonny wants more than to make a good living for himself. As the 2016 elections neared, he saw an opportunity for his people to get ahead of the game. The federal government was relaxing marijuana restrictions on tribal lands, granting the tribe some measure of autonomy over its marijuana policies. Sonny figured the Hoopa tribe could establish a foothold in the industry before legalization allows large-scale farms to dominate the industry.

In 2016, Sonny launched and financed a campaign to convince tribal members to support his vision for a revitalized Hoopa Valley agricultural community. He proposed construction of three ten-acre marijuana farms in the valley. The farms would employ tribal members, and return 50 percent of profits to the Hoopa Valley Tribe. Revenues would support education, employment, and rehabilitation programs that were sorely needed. A trust would be established to provide tuition funds to tribal members when they turn eighteen, funds would be dedicated to substance abuse counseling, and convicted felons would be given opportunities to develop their skills and establish a track record of employment.[9]

Perhaps the plan was too good to be true. Some tribal members were skeptical, and wondered if the scheme was an elaborate ruse for Sonny and Arthur to make a boatload of money. The tribe's educational community was concerned that the project would dissuade young people from finishing high school or going to college. And maybe having several marijuana farms on a reservation struggling with substance abuse would create too much temptation. Despite Sonny's best efforts, when it came time to cast ballots, the tribe rejected the proposal by eighty votes.

Shortly after the plan was defeated, California and several other states legalized recreational marijuana, and other tribes announced plans to develop marijuana farming operations. Sonny has since been approached by tribal members who have changed their minds and would support his proposal if given a second chance. But he isn't sure when the time will be right to push it again, or if he'll be up for another campaign.

"You see, the whole thing was, we were doing it for our grandkids," Sonny tells me. "I'm sixty-six. Arthur is sixty-three. We thought getting ahead on this would be ideal for our economy. For the reservation. They couldn't see the endgame where I was headed."

Arthur, too, is disappointed: "Everyone asked, 'What do *you* want out of this?' And I thought, we have the highest unemployment rate in the nation. I wanted people to have money to buy a car, to eat, to buy clothes. Otherwise, we got nothing here."

As our conversation continues, I get the impression Sonny is starting to talk himself into another run at his dream. I can tell he wants to leave a mark on the Hoopa Valley as his great-grandfather did before him. The marijuana farming collective, he knows, could revitalize the tribe's communal farming roots, creating a brighter future for his people.

"Here's the future for us here on the reservation," Sonny begins. "I believe what we're doing, if we can accomplish it, will eliminate the big businesses. This could be a preview of what farming should look like: owned and operated by Native Americans, and striving to have the best quality. We haven't given up, and we're not going to give up."

Writer Wendell Berry grew up on a tobacco farm in Henry County, Kentucky, in the 1930s and 40s. Tobacco, like many other crops, has increasingly been grown on fewer, larger farms, a trend that is just as true in Henry County as it is anywhere else. Berry appreciates more than most Americans what this transition to Big Agriculture looks like. In his 1977 book *The Unsettling of America*, Berry laments the deterioration of his family's farming community as the industry transitioned to Big Agriculture:

> In the decades since World War II the farms of Henry County have become increasingly mechanized. Though they are still comparatively diversified, they are less diversified than they used to be. The holdings are larger, the owners are fewer. The land is falling more and more into the hands of speculators and professional people from the cities, who—in spite of all the scientific agricultural miracles—still have much more money than the farmers. Because of big technology and big

economics, there is more abandoned land in the county than ever before. Many of the better farms are visibly deteriorating.[10]

In the years to come, when the federal marijuana prohibition is lifted and markets have their way with the farming community, will the same be said about Humboldt County? There is no shortage of suitors lining up to deliver a death blow to the tens of thousands of family farmers supplying the world with American marijuana. Big Agriculture. Big Tobacco. Big Pharmaceutical. Big Alcohol. Eventually, perhaps, Big Marijuana.

I have argued in this book that a Big Marijuana takeover is not inevitable; that the Big Marijuana prophecy is an empty forecast preying on our collective tendencies to think that bigger is always better when it comes to agriculture. But as Berry argues:

> As a social or economic goal, bigness is totalitarian; it establishes an inevitable tendency toward the *one* that will be the biggest of all. Many who got big to stay in are now being driven out by those who got bigger. The aim of bigness implies not one aim that is not socially and culturally destructive.
>
> And this community-killing agriculture, with its monomania of bigness, is not primarily the work of farmers, though it has burgeoned on their weaknesses. It is the work of the institutions of agriculture … who have promoted so-called efficiency at the expense of community (and of real efficiency), and quantity at the expense of quality.[11]

If proposals to protect and support small-scale marijuana farmers are rejected, any number of excuses would be provided. For example: Small farms are less efficient. Small farms raise prices for consumers. Small farms are classist. Small farms are harder to regulate. Small farms don't produce uniform marijuana. Small farms feed the black market. Small farms can't compete.

There will be those who say that if small farms can't survive in a free market economy, well, then, that's their fault. Such a claim would be inaccurate and ultimately beside the point. All across North America, states are creating artificial monopolies or oligopolies that give moneyed interests control over production, or at least a head start. Canada issued a contract to a single company to supply the entire country's legal medical marijuana market. Florida and New York, the third and fourth most populous states, respectively, issued cultivation licenses to less than a dozen companies, many of which were politically connected. And Ohio's failed 2015 legalization initiative was shameless on its face—the companies funding the legalization campaign tried to give themselves a monopoly on production by inserting their names and exclusive cultivation rights into the state's constitution.

States that promote bigness do so at their peril. There are many reasons family farms represent the ideal agricultural foundation for the marijuana industry. This book has been, in part, an attempt to identify and explore those reasons. But there is one final reason that I've been dancing around (though it has been an implicit theme throughout this book)—marijuana agriculture may present a once-in-a-lifetime opportunity to spark the rebirth of the American family farm.

As marijuana rises on the list of America's largest cash crops, so too does the influence of the marijuana farming community. This community is no longer a social, political, and economic outcast. On the contrary, marijuana farmers are claiming their place in the hierarchy of American agriculture. Perhaps that position will be short-lived, forgotten as soon as Big Marijuana claims the industry's seat at America's economic table.

But what if it isn't short-lived? What if billions of dollars of consumer spending is channeled into small-scale, diversified, local, organic family farms? The marijuana industry has more than enough capital to lead an agrarian renaissance, so why not take advantage? Which state isn't interested in creating new jobs in underserved rural areas? Which state isn't interested in attracting the next generation of farmers to their struggling communities?

It might be possible to grow the entire country's supply of marijuana on a few very large farms. But whose interests would that serve? Not the states and counties that lost out on agricultural development. Not the family farmers who can't make a living and are forced to move to urban centers. Not the consumers who just saw thousands of product choices disappear before their eyes. The only interests a Big Marijuana model serves is Big Marijuana itself—"the *one* that will be the biggest of all."

Berry pleaded over forty years ago that time was running out to save our rural communities:

A healthy *farm* culture can be based only upon familiarity and can grow only among a people soundly established upon the land; it nourishes and it safe-guards a human intelligence of the earth that no amount of technology can satisfactorily replace. The growth of such a culture was once a strong possibility in the farm communities of this country. We now have only the sad remnants of those communities. If we allow another generation to pass without doing what is necessary to enhance and embolden the possibility now perishing with them, we will lose it altogether. And then we will not only invoke calamity—we will deserve it.[12]

For the past decade or so, Americans have struggled to address a growing dissatisfaction with the state of food and agriculture in this country.

An agricultural model dependent on monocultural production, chemical inputs, and global transportation presents few wins for consumers. Price-sensitive consumers who benefit from rock-bottom food prices end up paying the long-term costs of malnutrition. Discerning consumers have limited means of supporting local family farms, and the lack of regulation of high-end grocery store products does not inspire confidence.[13]

Despite these concerns, not much has been done to change the agricultural model that leaves so many Americans wanting. In part, that's because Big Agriculture has a large stake in the status quo, and is working diligently to prevent it from being disrupted. Even when the general public approaches consensus on a problem such as this one, the problem will always be difficult to address if powerful economic forces are willing to do everything in their power to make sure the solutions don't change the factual realities.

But consider: that isn't the case for marijuana agriculture—or at least not yet. The marijuana farming community is still predominantly composed of family farmers. There is very little standing in the way of a public effort to create an agricultural model for the marijuana industry that represents the public interest. Of course, there isn't yet a consensus on what constitutes the public interest—but at least there's an opportunity for Americans to take matters into their own hands. The marijuana industry is begging to be shaped by the people. In some cases policymakers have literally begged for assistance. Why not give it to them?

Keith Stroup has been providing assistance to policymakers since 1970. Stroup grew up on a family farm in southern Illinois, in a poor, rural part of the state. The farm was located right outside of Dix, Illinois, a sleepy town of around 200 farmers and coal miners. The Stroup farm grew corn and soybeans and raised a flock of sheep. Stroup describes his childhood on the farm as a "happy environment," but by the time he graduated from the University of Illinois, he couldn't wait to get out of the Midwest.

Stroup moved to Washington D.C., to attend law school, and started working in the same circles as Ralph Nader. Nader encouraged him to advocate for the repeal of marijuana prohibition. In hindsight, Stroup was just the right person for the job: he was young and bright, and plugged into the anti-Vietnam War movement, which was also sympathetic to marijuana legalization. In 1970, Stroup founded the National Organization for the

Repeal of Marijuana Laws (NORML). He's been fighting for an end to marijuana prohibition ever since.

NORML typically takes a consumer perspective on marijuana legalization and regulation issues, rather than a farmer's perspective. So I figured Stroup would be just the right person to talk to in order to find out what consumers are saying about the Big Marijuana prophecy.

"I don't think I've ever had anyone approach me that said, 'Boy, I wish Big Tobacco would just take over,'" he told me. "The culture has generally accepted common principles: smaller is better, and local is better, and organic is better. And I'm delighted with all of those tendencies. I do think that's important to consumers."

Can consumers and farmers work together to keep marijuana farming small, sustainable, and local? Stroup believes they can. In fact, preserving the right of the people to grow marijuana at home for personal use may be the key to bridging the divide between consumers and family farmers. "If the market tries to sell us marijuana that's too weak, or not good quality, then to hell with it! We'll grow our own," Stroup said. At-home cultivation might also give consumers an appreciation for their local family farmers—growing isn't as easy as it looks.

But Stroup is aware of the danger that Big Marijuana presents. He's starting to see bigger players jockey for position as the legalization movement picks up steam. That hasn't always created the best outcome for consumers or family farmers. "In Florida, you talk about the limited number of [licensed marijuana] producers down there. That was the most corrupt thing ever," he says. "Obviously, you're creating a cartel if you only allow a few people to control the industry."

Thankfully the Florida approach is still the minority approach. In other states that are more inclusive, Stroup sees the marijuana industry as a boon to family farmers. "Once it gets legalized, I think you'll see all kinds of small farmers welcome the opportunity to have another crop," he suggested. "And culturally, it will be nice for a lot of those traditional farmers to reexamine their views on marijuana and realize we're all neighbors."

Stroup's colleague Crystal Oliver is active in the Washington State chapter of NORML. She has been emphasizing to legislators and the farming community the economic benefits of marijuana farming for local communities, especially when factoring in the relatively small acreage being used to cultivate marijuana. When Crystal presented preliminary data on marijuana farm revenues per acre, other farmers were stunned. "Wheat farmers in Spokane County grossed $62 million in revenues last year. Marijuana farmers grossed $63 million. When I told them all those marijuana revenues were generated on less than fifty acres, the room went quiet."

Crystal also talks about the demographic imperative of developing the next generation of family farmers. "Here in Washington, the average marijuana farmer is in their thirties, which is over twenty years younger than the average non-marijuana farmer," she pointed out. If the American family farm is going to survive, young people will need to be willing to live in the country and work the land. Marijuana might be the plant that can get them there.

Looking to the future, there will inevitably be conflicts within the marijuana farming community, especially as the legalization movement proceeds and legal markets mature and go through their growing pains. The key for getting through these tough times is to remember that many marijuana farmers are part of a meaningful, positive, and growing farming community, and that community is an essential part of the broader community of the American people. We gain from cooperation much more than we lose. Berry observed this as well:

> If a culture is to hope for any longevity, then the relationships within it must, in recognition of their interdependence, be predominantly cooperative rather than competitive. A people cannot live long at each other's expense or at the expense of their cultural birthright—just as an agriculture cannot live long at the expense of its soil or its work force, and just as in a natural system the competitions among species must be limited if all are to survive.[14]

Working on this book has introduced me to many thoughtful, passionate people concerned about the future of the marijuana industry. Almost all of them have stressed the need for the community to set aside its differences and work together during these hectic and unpredictable days of legalization. From Joy Beckerman and Courtney Moran extending an olive branch on behalf of the hemp community, to Sonny Jackson urging the Hoopa tribe to create a farming cooperative, opportunities to form partnerships will continue to present themselves. If small-scale farmers are going to survive the inevitable onslaught of bigness, the marijuana community will need to come together to create something even bigger.

I opened this book with my friend Jack and his farm. Jack and I have been friends for a long time. Like any relationship, ours has waxed and waned, with long absences bridging some of my life's fondest memories. When Jack bought his farm several years ago, I was surprised to feel so drawn to his land. The farm is more than a row of marijuana crops and a few acres of grapes; it has become my shrine to the agrarian ideal.

Sometimes, admittedly, reality falls short of the romantic image I hold in my head. During one of my visits, Jack and his crew spent an entire week picking rocks out of a field and piling them in a corner. For several weeks in August of 2017, residual smoke from nearby wildfires was so thick it wasn't safe to breathe outside. And the marijuana business still attracts some unsavory characters on occasion.

But it's hard for me to overstate the thrill I get watching my friend come into his own as a man, a farmer, a boss, and a pillar of his community. Wildfires wiped out Jack's grape harvest in 2017, but the late-season marijuana crops produced big, healthy, good-looking yields. It was the kind of harvest Jack needed to launch him into another year of new projects and big plans.

Now that his farm is running smoothly, Jack is looking to take his business to the next level. It can be difficult to sell marijuana in Humboldt County, the epicenter of the American marijuana farming community. Jack is a capable negotiator, but after a few weeks of lowball offers, he was eager to see what else he could get. So he took some samples of his best strains and drove twelve hours south, to the sprawling metropolis of Los Angeles. Jack was introduced to dispensary owners and big-time distributors, making connections and gaining valuable inside information.

It was an eye-opening experience for him. He told me, "Humboldt can be so ... Humboldt. Sometimes you lose sight of what's going on out there in the rest of the world." It's not easy for either of us to know what the future holds for the marijuana industry. Will Big Marijuana wipe out small farms like Jack's, or will family farmers band together to take down Goliath? Can indoor and outdoor farmers push each other to new heights? Can marijuana and hemp farmers coexist? Can regulators and farmers work together?

There's a future for marijuana agriculture; that much is clear. And I believe family farms can be that future if the American people and the farming community want it to happen.

Wendell Berry might respond to this belief not by refuting it, but by pointing out that I am feeding into what he calls the "cult of the future," a modern obsession with the future that obscures what is happening in the present: "It is no doubt impossible to live without thought of the future; hope and vision can live nowhere else. But the only possible guarantee of the future is responsible behavior in the present."[15]

I can't think of a more responsible approach to marijuana agriculture than a vigorous and cooperative community of family farms, supplying consumers with sustainable, high-quality marijuana, right here in the U.S.A.

Notes

Chapter 1

1. Nina Shapiro, "How Jamen Shively's Big Marijuana Boast Went South," *Seattle Weekly News*, October 8, 2014, accessed January 11, 2018, http://goo.gl/HB6c0e.

2. "Jamen Shively Biography," *Medical Jane*, accessed on August 1, 2016, https://goo.gl/CQxP0y.

3. Quoted in Mike Riggs, "Former Microsoft Employee Plans to Be the Bill Gates of Weed," *Hit & Run Blog*, Reason.com, May 29, 2013, accessed January 11, 2018, http://goo.gl/Ukyzl7.

4. Quoted in Tony Dokoupil, "Vice Wars: Tobacco, Alcohol and the Rise of Big Marijuana," NBC News, November 29, 2014, accessed January 11, 2018, http://goo.gl/CrXqSB.

5. Quoted in Trevor Hughes, "Will Big Tobacco Become Big Marijuana?" *USA Today*, April 11, 2015, accessed on January 11, 2018, http://goo.gl/6MSugh.

6. Rachel Ann Barry, Heikki Hiilamo, and Stanton A. Glantz, "Waiting for the Opportune Moment: The Tobacco Industry and Marijuana Legalization," *Milbank Quarterly* 92, no. 2 (June 2014).

7. Quoted in "The Challenge of 'Big Marijuana,'" *Christian Science Monitor*, March 7, 2016, https://www.csmonitor.com/Commentary/the-monitors-view/2016/0307/The-challenge-of-Big-Marijuana.

8. Charlie Baker, Maura Healey, and Marty Walsh, "Mass. Should Not Legalize Marijuana," *Boston Globe*, March 4, 2016, accessed January 11, 2018, https://goo.gl/MVJRGT. (Recreational marijuana was, however, legalized in Massachusetts by ballot initiative later in 2016.)

9. The bill's summary begins, "Relates to the medical use of marihuana; legalizes the possession, manufacture, use, delivery, transport or administration of medical marihuana by a designated caregiver for a certified medical use." Compassionate

Care Act, New York State Assembly: A06357 (2015–2016); *New York Codes, Rules and Regulations*, vol. D, Title 10, chapter 13—"Medical Use of Marihuana."

10. "Manufacturing of medical marihuana by a registered organization shall only be done in an indoor, enclosed, secure facility located in New York State, which may include a greenhouse." New York Health and Safety Code §3364(8).

11. Task Force on the Implementation of Amendment 64, *Regulation of Marijuana in Colorado* (State of Colorado, 2013), 64, http://hermes.cde.state.co.us/drupal/is landora/object/co%3A11782/datastream/OBJ/view.

12. Quoted in Hughes, "Will Big Tobacco Become Big Marijuana?"

13. Quoted in Tim Fernholz, "Temptation Goods: America's Weed Industry Is Going to Be Massive. Is Big Marijuana a Good Thing?," *Quartz*, April 20, 2016, accessed January 18, 2018, https://qz.com/664956/americas-weed-industry-is-going-to-be -massive-is-big-marijuana-a-good-thing/.

14. Steering Committee, Blue Ribbon Commission on Marijuana Policy, *Pathways Report: Policy Options for Regulating Marijuana in California* (California, 2015), https:// www.sfchronicle.com/file/110/4/1104-BRCReportJuly20-FINAL.pdf.

15. James MacDonald, Penni Korb, and Robert Hoppe, *Farm Size and the Organization of U.S. Crop Farming*, USDA Economic Research Report 152 (August 2013), accessed January 11, 2018, http://goo.gl/e8Tdwl.

16. Colorado Senator Chris Holbert, quoted in Kristen Wyatt, "Legalized States Taking a Fresh Look at Out-of-State Marijuana Investing," *Cannabist*, January 20, 2016, accessed January 11, 2018, http://goo.gl/9Dz5S0.

17. Rick Anderson, "How New Rules in Two States Could Give Birth to Big Marijuana," *Los Angeles Times*, March 24, 2016, accessed January 11, 2018, http://goo.gl/HA5BBb.

18. Quoted in Dokoupil, "Vice Wars."

19. Deborah Bonello, "Mexican Marijuana Farmers See Profits Tumble as U.S. Loos-ens Laws," *Los Angeles Times*, December 30, 2015, accessed January 11, 2018, http:// goo.gl/udEjtG.

20. Christopher Ingraham, "Legal Marijuana Is Finally Doing What the Drug War Couldn't," *Washington Post*, March 3, 2016, accessed January 11, 2018, https://goo.gl /P7Noy6.

21. U.S. Department of Justice Drug Enforcement Administration, *2015 National Drug Threat Assessment Summary* (October 2015), https://goo.gl/kr1toR, 71.

22. Ibid.

23. Nick Miroff, "Losing Marijuana Business, Mexican Cartels Push Heroin and Meth," *Washington Post*, January 11, 2015, accessed January 11, 2018, https://goo.gl/L18tuw.

24. Steven Nelson, "DEA: Cartels Now Smuggle U.S. Pot into Mexico," *US News & World Report*, December 2, 2014, accessed January 11, 2018, http://goo.gl/5ZWKEx.

25. Hans Taparia and Pamela Koch, "A Seismic Shift in How People Eat," *New York Times*, November 6, 2015, accessed January 11, 2018, http://goo.gl/vKt7j5.

26. "Preventing Big Tobacco 2.0," Smart Approaches to Marijuana," accessed January 16, 2018, https://learnaboutsam.org/.

27. Evan Mills, "The Carbon Footprint of Indoor Cannabis Production," *Energy Consumption* 46 (2012): 59.

28. Jennifer Oldham, "As Pot-Growing Expands, Electricity Demands Tax U.S. Grids," *Bloomberg*, December 21, 2015, accessed January 11, 2018, http://goo.gl/JO0dte.

29. Scott Bauer et al., "Impacts of Surface Water Diversions for Marijuana Cultivation on Aquatic Habitat in Four Northwestern California Watersheds," *PLOS One* 10, no. 9 (2015): 3, accessed January 11, 2018, https://doi.org/10.1371/journal.pone.0120016.

30. Andrew Goff, "Major Multi-Agency Marijuana Raid in Island Mountain Today," *Local Coast Outpost*, June 22, 2015, accessed January 11, 2018, http://goo.gl/Ga8iZs.

31. Adam Randall, "Tri-county Pot Raids Net 86,578 Plants," *Ukiah Daily Journal*, June 29, 2015, accessed January 11, 2018, http://goo.gl/5h2HWZ.

32. Quoted in Wil S. Hylton, "Willie Nelson's Crusade to Stop Big Pot," *New York*, November 1, 2015.

33. See generally Rowan Robinson, *The Great Book of Hemp: The Complete Guide to the Environmental, Commercial, and Medicinal Uses of the World's Most Extraordinary Plant* (Rochester, VA: Park Street Press, 1996).

Chapter 2

1. Ted Goebel, "The Missing Years for Modern Humans," *Science* 315, no. 5809 (January 2007): 194, http://www.jstor.org/stable/20035192.

2. Clive Finlayson, *The Improbable Primate: How Water Shaped Human Evolution* (New York: Oxford University Press, 2014).

3. Goebel, "The Missing Years for Modern Humans," 194–196.

4. Terence A. Brown, Martin K. Jones, Wayne Powell, and Robin G. Allaby, "The Complex Origins of Domesticated Crops in the Fertile Crescent," *Trends in Ecology and Evolution* 24, no. 2 (February 2009): 103–109.

5. Robert Clarke and Mark Merlin, *Cannabis: Evolution and Ethnobotany* (Berkeley: University of California Press, 2013).

6. Hui-Lin Li, "The Origin and Use of Cannabis in Eastern Asia: Linguistic-Cultural Implications," *Economic Botany* 28, no. 3 (July 1974): 293–301.

7. Clarke and Merlin, *Cannabis*, 77.

8. Ibid., citing Nikolai Vavilov.

9. David E. Newton, *Marijuana: A Reference Handbook*, 2nd ed. (Santa Barbara, CA: ABC-CLIO, 2017), 3; Clarke and Merlin, *Cannabis*, 142–143.

10. Clarke and Merlin, *Cannabis*, 143, citing Nicholas Tarling, *The Cambridge History of Southeast Asia*, vol. 1, *From Early Times to c. 1500* (New York: Cambridge University Press, 1999).

11. Ibid., citing J. G. Andersson, "An Early Chinese Culture," *Bulletin of Geological Survey of China*, no. 5 (Peking, Ministry of Agriculture and Commerce, 1923); see also Martin Booth, *Cannabis: A History* (New York: St. Martin's Press, 2005).

12. Clarke and Merlin, *Cannabis*, 138.

13. Booth, *Cannabis: A History*, 19.

14. Ibid., 20.

15. Ibid., 21.

16. Ibid., 22.

17. Clarke and Merlin, *Cannabis*, 339.

18. Booth, *Cannabis: A History*, 26.

19. Ibid.

20. Ibid., 31.

21. Ibid., 30.

22. Clarke and Merlin, *Cannabis*, 342.

23. Wool Act 1699, Kingdom of England, British History Online, accessed March 15, 2018, http://www.british-history.ac.uk/statutes-realm/vol7/pp600-602.

24. Letter from George Washington to William Pearce, May 29, 1796, Founders Online (National Archives, last modified June 29, 2017), https://founders.archives.gov/documents/Washington/99-01-02-00559.

25. Humphrey Ploughjogger (pseudonym of John Adams) to the *Boston Evening-Post*, June 20, 1763, in *Papers of John Adams*, ed. Robert J. Taylor et al., vol. 1 (Cambridge, MA: Belknap Press of Harvard University Press, 1977), 63, 66.

26. Quoted in Rowan Robinson, *The Great Book of Hemp: The Complete Guide to the Environmental, Commercial, and Medicinal Uses of the World's Most Extraordinary Plant* (Rochester, VT: Park Street Press, 1996).

27. Booth, *Cannabis: A History*, 36.

28. Clarke and Merlin, *Cannabis*, 591.

29. Booth, *Cannabis: A History*, 121.

30. Clarke and Merlin, *Cannabis*, 605–606.

31. Jonathon Green, *Cannabis* (New York: Thunder's Mouth Press, 2002).

32. Jack Herer, *The Emperor Wears No Clothes*, 12th ed. (Van Nuys, CA: Ah Ha Publishing, 2011), 24.

33. Booth, *Cannabis: A History*, 19.

34. Ibid., 39.

35. Clarke and Merlin, *Cannabis*, 233, quoting L. Lewin, *Phantastica* (New York: E. P. Dutton, 1964).

36. Michael Pollan, *The Botany of Desire* (New York: Random House, 2001), 173–175.

37. Clarke and Merlin, *Cannabis*, 340.

38. Ibid., 617–618.

39. David Bewley-Taylor, Tom Blickman, and Martin Jelsma, *The Rise and Decline of Cannabis Prohibition: The History of Cannabis in the UN Drug Control System and Options for Reform*, Transnational Institute and Global Drug Policy Observatory (Amsterdam, 2014), 6.

40. Clarke and Merlin, *Cannabis*, 618.

41. Bewley-Taylor, Blickman, and Jelsma, *The Rise and Decline of Cannabis Prohibition*, 6.

42. Clarke and Merlin, *Cannabis*, 619–620.

43. Quoted in DJ Guba, "Chapter 2—French Creoles in Egypt: Jacques 'Abdallah' Menou and France's First Anti-Drug Law," Academia.edu, accessed January 11, 2018, https://www.academia.edu/22614867/Chapter_2_-_French_Creoles_in_Egypt_Jacques_Abdallah_Menou_and_Frances_First_Anti-Drug_Law.

44. David A. Guba, "Antoine Isaac Silvestre de Sacy and the Myth of the Hachichins: Orientalizing Hashish in Nineteenth-Century France," *Social History of Alcohol and Drugs* 30 (2016): 50–74.

45. Booth, *Cannabis: A History*, 66–75.

46. Ibid., 22.

47. Quoted in ibid., 59–60.

48. Ibid., 61.

49. Danilo Balotta, Henri Bergeron, and Brendan Hughes, "Cannabis Control in Europe," in *A Cannabis Reader: Global Issues and Local Experiences*, 8 EMCDDA 1 (2008): 100; Bewley-Taylor, Blickman, and Jelsma, *The Rise and Decline of Cannabis Prohibition*, 7.

50. *Report of the Indian Hemp Drugs Commission*, 1894–1895, vol. 1, http://digital.nls .uk/indiapapers/browse/archive/74574854.

51. Ibid.

52. Ibid.

53. Booth, *Cannabis: A History*, 115.

54. Clarke and Merlin, *Cannabis*, 617.

Chapter 3

1. Nixon Tapes, Conversation 505-4, Meeting between Nixon and H. R. "Bob" Haldeman, May 26, 1971, transcript available at Common Sense for Drug Policy, accessed March 15, 2018, http://www.csdp.org/research/nixonpot.txt.

2. Most of the marijuana grown outdoors in northern California is harvested in the fall, when prices are at their lowest. If a farmer can afford to wait until late winter or spring when the market's supply is diminished, the payoff can be substantial. Prices increase further if the farmer is willing to transport the harvest herself. Generally speaking, the further you get from Humboldt County (where marijuana is ubiquitous), the more you'll earn. Of course, both the "wait-until-spring" and "deliver-yourself" strategies carry added risk.

3. A farmer growing high-quality marijuana still gets the most value from selling marijuana buds in their raw form (nowadays a farmer is expected to dry and trim the buds himself prior to sale). Even the highest-quality crops have some inconsistency, however, and some buds will be less marketable, either because of their size (buds that are too small or too big frustrate the uniformity of the pounds being sold), composition (such as a disproportionately high percentage of leaves, twigs, or seeds), treatment (poorly harvested, trimmed, or stored), or some other factor. These lower-grade buds can still be packaged together and sold for a low, uninspiring price. Or, with a little effort, the farmer can put together a makeshift hash lab to produce hash oil by

extracting the THC from the bud (the THC content is often just as high regardless of the grade of the bud). The hash oil can then be sold for a more satisfactory price. A hash lab requires significant start-up costs, naturally, as well as expertise. In California, producing hash oil also requires an additional license.

4. *Cultivation: Capitalizing on a Tripling of Legal Demand*, Cannabis Intelligence Briefing series, 5th ed. (Arcview Market Research, 2017).

5. *The State of Legal Marijuana Markets*, 5th ed. (Arcview Market Research, 2017).

6. "The Piercing Words of James Baldwin," Biography.com, August 1, 2017, accessed January 16, 2018, https://www.biography.com/news/james-baldwin-quotes.

7. Cited in Martin Booth, *Cannabis: A History* (New York: St. Martin's Press, 2005), 164.

8. "There is no evidence that Marihuana [sic] as grown and used is a habit-forming drug ... or that it has any appreciable deleterious influence on the individual using it." Panama Canal Zone Governor's Committee, April–December 1925, in *The Military Surgeon*, Journal of the Association of Military Surgeons of the United States (November 1933), 274.

9. Jazz musicians of the era quickly discovered that a cerebral marijuana high pairs well with the free-form, improvisational nature of jazz. Hoagy Carmichael described this sensation while playing with Louis Armstrong: "the muggles took effect and my body got light. Every note Louis hit was perfection ... I had never heard the tune before, but somehow I couldn't miss. I was floating in a strange deep blue whirlpool of jazz." Quoted in Nat Shapiro and Nat Hentoff, *Hear Me Talkin' to Ya: The Story of Jazz as Told by the Men Who Made It* (New York: Dover, 1966), 142.

10. The perpetrators of these crimes were almost always depicted as Mexican or African-American, while the victims were almost always white.

11. Quoted in Jack Herer, *The Emperor Wears No Clothes*, 12th ed. (Van Nuys, CA: Ah Ha Publishing, 2011), 59.

12. Ibid., 57.

13. Ibid., 52.

14. Richard J. Bonnie and Charles H. Whitebread, "The Forbidden Fruit and the Tree of Knowledge: An Inquiry into the Legal History of American Marijuana Prohibition," 56 *Virginia Law Review* 971 (1970).

15. At the same time, though, *Time* magazine noted the existence of a cottage industry of small-scale American growers: "It can be grown easily almost anywhere ... but its furtive preparation and sale provide a modest living to thousands." "Music: The Weed," *Time*, July 19, 1943.

16. Booth, *Cannabis: A History*, 159. Farmers were incentivized to grow hemp with generous subsidies and an exemption from military service.

17. Martin A. Lee, *Smoke Signals: A Social History of Marijuana—Medical, Recreational, and Scientific* (New York: Scribner, 2012), 65. The *New York Times* noted during the Cold War that, in the fight for hearts and minds around the world, "America's secret weapon is a blue note in a minor key [and] its most effective ambassador is Louis Armstrong." Felix Belair Jr., "United States Has Secret Sonic Weapon—Jazz," *New York Times*, November 6, 1955.

18. Lee, *Smoke Signals*, 78.

19. This line is attributed to Jack Weinberg; see Paul Galloway, "Radical Redux," *Chicago Tribune*, November 11, 2016, accessed January 11, 2018, http://articles .chicagotribune.com/1990-11-16/features/9004050125_1_jack-weinberg-california -gubernatorial-candidate-berkeley.

20. These buds are what are bought and sold as raw marijuana, or "flower."

21. Booth, *Cannabis: A History*, 228–230.

22. Ibid., 232.

23. Ibid., 235.

24. Lee, *Smoke Signals*, 117–118.

25. Booth, *Cannabis: A History*, 234.

26. Lee, *Smoke Signals*, 151.

27. Ibid., 149.

28. The Supreme Court reasoned that, because compliance with the act required a possessor of marijuana to identify himself or herself as a member of a "selective group inherently suspect of criminal activities," the act created a "real and appreciable" hazard of self-incrimination, a violation of the Fifth Amendment of the Constitution. *Leary v. United States*, 395 U.S. 6, 18 (1969).

29. Under normal circumstances, border agents would conduct a three-minute search of every twentieth vehicle.

30. Lee, *Smoke Signals*, 116.

31. G. Gordon Liddy, *Will: The Autobiography of G. Gorgon Liddy* (New York: St. Martin's Press, 1997), 135.

32. Notably, Operation Intercept was endorsed by the governor of California, Ronald Reagan.

33. Christopher Rose, host, "Episode 66: Operation Intercept," *15 Minute History*, podcast audio, March 25, 2015, accessed January 11, 2018, https://15minutehistory .org/2015/03/25/episode-66-operation-intercept/.

34. Edward Jay Epstein, "Operation Intercept," chapter 7 of *Agency of Fear: Opiates and Political Power in America*, Schaffer Library of Drug Policy, accessed March 19, 2018, http://www.druglibrary.org/schaffer/history/aof/AOF7.html.

35. Lawrence A. Gooberman, "Operation Intercept: The Multiple Consequences of Public Policy" (Pergamon Press, 1974), Schaffer Library of Drug Policy, accessed January 11, 2018, http://www.druglibrary.org/schaffer/history/e1960/intercept/default.htm.

36. "Pot: Year of the Famine," *Newsweek*, September 22, 1969, 37.

37. A few months later, to smooth things over, Nixon agreed to cede to Mexico the majority of a parcel of land in (or near, depending on your perspective) west Texas that had been in dispute.

38. Cocaine and methamphetamine were classified as Schedule II drugs on the grounds that they have medicinal value.

39. David T. Courtwright, "The Controlled Substances Act: How a 'Big Tent' Reform Became a Punitive Drug Law," *Drug and Alcohol Dependence* 76, no. 1 (October 5, 2004), https://doi.org/10.1016/j.drugalcdep.2004.04.012.

40. Booth, *Cannabis: A History*, 241.

41. Ibid., 245.

42. Caroline M. Tanner et al., "Rotenone, Paraquat, and Parkinson's Disease," *Environmental Health Perspectives* 119, no. 6 (June 2011): 866–872, accessed January 11, 2018, https://www.ncbi.nlm.nih.gov/pmc/articles/PMC3114824.

43. PAN Germany, "Paraquat and Suicide—2013 Fact Sheet," http://www.pan-germany .org/download/_paraquat2.pdf.

44. Booth, *Cannabis: A History*, 251.

45. Ibid., 252.

46. Ronald Chepesiuk, *The Bullet or the Bribe: Taking Down Colombia's Cali Drug Cartel* (Santa Barbara, CA: Praeger Publishers, 2003), 23–26.

47. By one estimate, American marijuana farmers claimed a 15 percent share of the domestically consumed market by 1982.

48. Lee, *Smoke Signals*, 174.

49. Associated Press, "U.S. to Resume Using Paraquat on Marijuana," *New York Times*, July 14, 1988, accessed January 11, 2018, http://www.nytimes.com/1988/07 /14/us/us-to-resume-using-paraquat-on-marijuana.html.

50. Federal institutions participating in CAMP included the U.S. Coast Guard; Marshals Service; Forest Service; Internal Revenue Service; Bureau of Alcohol, Tobacco, and Firearms; and Customs and Border Protection. State agencies that participated included the California Bureau of Land Management, Department of Fish and Game, Department of Forestry, Department of Corrections, and the Highway Patrol. County sheriff's offices were also involved.

51. Dominic Corva, "Requiem for a CAMP: The Life and Death of a Domestic U.S. Drug War Institution," *International Journal of Drug Policy* 25, no. 1 (January 2014): 74.

52. CAMP was shut down in 2012.

53. Quoted in Corva, "Requiem for a CAMP," 78.

54. Ibid., 74.

55. Lee, *Smoke Signals*, 174.

56. United States Department of Justice, *Central Valley California High Intensity Drug Trafficking Area: Drug Market Analysis 2010*, https://www.justice.gov/archive/ndic/pubs40/40384/40384p.pdf; and Corva, "Requiem for a CAMP," 72.

57. Anecdotal evidence suggests the price for a pound of marijuana stayed relatively constant throughout the early CAMP years: around $4,000.

58. Corva, "Requiem for a CAMP," 74.

59. However, whatever violence did exist in the marijuana farming community in the United States may have been exaggerated by CAMP and the DEA.

60. Cocaine and heroin use rose sharply in the 1980s, accompanied by a rise in violent crime and robberies.

61. Ray Raphael, *Cash Crop: An American Dream* (Caspar, CA: Ridge Times Press, 1985), 171.

Chapter 4

1. "October 6, 1996, Presidential Debate with Senator Bob Dole," President Bill Clinton and Senator Bob Dole, University of Virginia Mill Center Presidential Speeches of Bill Clinton Presidency, accessed January 11, 2018, https://millercenter.org/the-presidency/presidential-speeches/october-6-1996-presidential-debate-senator-bob-dole.

2. Mollie Reilly, "Bill Clinton: 'There's a Lot of Evidence' in Favor of Legal Medical Marijuana," *Huffington Post*, June 29, 2014, accessed January 11, 2018, https://www.huffingtonpost.com/2014/06/29/bill-clinton-medical-marijuana_n_5541423.html.

3. This type of name isn't particularly unusual for Humboldt County.

4. Medical Marijuana Program, California Health and Safety Code §11362.5 (2017).

5. Regulate Marijuana Like Alcohol Act, Colorado Constitution, Article XVIII, Section 16 (2012) (Colorado Constitutional amendment 64); On Marijuana Reform, Washington Initiative Measure 502 (2012).

6. "29 Legal Medical Marijuana States and DC," ProCon.org, November 30, 2017, accessed January 12, 2018, https://medicalmarijuana.procon.org/view.resource.php ?resourceID=000881&print=true. "Marijuana Overview: Legalization," National Conference of State Legislatures, August 30, 2017, accessed January 12, 2018, http://www.ncsl.org/research/civil-and-criminal-justice/marijuana-overview.aspx.

7. By "strict prohibition policy," I mean states that have passed neither decriminalization laws nor allow for nonpsychoactive marijuana consumption for medical purposes. These states are Idaho, Kansas, and South Dakota. See "Marijuana Overview: Legalization"; "State Medical Marijuana Laws," National Conference of State Legislatures, September 14, 2017, accessed January 12, 2018, http://www.ncsl.org /research/health/state-medical-marijuana-laws.aspx.

8. According to the U.S. Census Bureau's July 2016 estimates, the combined population of Idaho, Kansas, and South Dakota is 5,455,883, while the estimated population of the United States is 323,127,513. "Quick Facts," Population Estimates, July 1, 2016, United States Census Bureau, accessed on October 16, 2017, https://goo.gl/zlyP5G.

9. Alex Kreit, "The 2015 Federal Budget's Medical Marijuana Provision: An 'End to the Federal Ban on Marijuana' or Something Less Than That?," *Northern Illinois University Law Review* 35, no. 537 (2015).

10. Aviva Shen, "The DEA Is Still Clinging to Reagan-Era Hysteria over Marijuana," *Think Progress*, August 11, 2016, https://thinkprogress.org/the-dea-is-still-clinging-to -the-war-on-drugs-417a4982bfd8/.

11. Jennifer DePinto, Fred Backus, Kabir Khanna, and Anthony Salvanto, "Marijuana Legalization Support at All-Time-High," CBS News, April 20, 2017, https:// www.cbsnews.com/news/support-for-marijuana-legalization-at-all-time-high/.

12. *New State Ice Co. v. Liebmann*, 285 U.S. 262 (1932).

13. Noelle Crombie, "Legal Marijuana in Oregon: A Look at the State's Pot History," *Oregonian*, November 7, 2014, http://www.oregonlive.com/marijuana/index.ssf /2014/11/legal_marijuana_in_oregon_a_lo.html.

14. According to one study, by 2010 nearly 80 percent of the marijuana consumed in the United States came from California. Emily Brady, "How Humboldt Became America's Marijuana Capital," *Salon*, June 30, 2013, http://goo.gl/529p1p.

15. Medical Marijuana Program Act, S.B. 420 §11362.77 (2013).

16. Ibid.

17. *People v. Kelly*, 77 Cal. Rptr. 3d 390 (Cal. 2010).

18. Alissa Walker, "How Growing More Weed Can Help California Fix Its Water Problems," *Gizmodo*, October 12, 2015, http://goo.gl/ZEwFpT.

19. Ibid.

20. Medical Marijuana, California Senate Bill No. 643, Chapter 719 (Deering 2015).

21. Medical Marijuana Regulation and Safety Act, California Statute AB No. 243 §19332(a-e).

22. "Assembly Members Urge Governor Brown to Sign Medical Marijuana Package," News Channel 3, KIEM TV, accessed on October 16, 2017, https://perma.cc/K4D7 -WY6L.

23. *Task Force Report on the Implementation of Amendment 64: Regulation of Marijuana in Colorado*, State of Colorado (2013).

24. Bryce Pardo, "Cannabis Policy Reforms in the Americas: A Comparative Analysis of Colorado, Washington and Uruguay," *International Journal of Drug Policy* 25, no. 4 (July 2014): 727; also see Implementing Retail Marijuana, Colorado House Bill 13-1318, Colorado Session 69 (2013). The task force's recommendations were largely adopted by the state legislature and passed in May 2013; see Implementing Retail Marijuana, House Bill 13-1317, Senate Bill 283, Colorado Session 69 (2013).

25. *Task Force Report on the Implementation of Amendment 64*.

26. Washington State Liquor and Cannabis Board, homepage, accessed on October 16, 2017, http://goo.gl/k8V72J.

27. Compassionate Medical Cannabis Act of 2014, Florida Senate Bill 1030 (2014).

28. Medical Use of Marijuana, New York Assembly Bill A06357 (2014); see also Catherine Rafter, "New York State Just Granted Five Medical Marijuana Licenses," *Observer*, July 31, 2015, http://goo.gl/JqBdtG.

29. In principle, states can tailor any number of water or agricultural permits, but there is a limit to how extensive the specifications can be when administering large volumes of permit applications; see Gary D. Lynne, J. S. Shonkwiler, and Michael E. Wilson, "Water Permitting Behavior under the 1972 Florida Water Resources Act," *Land Economics* 67, no. 3 (1991): 340, http://www.jstor.org/stable/3146429.

30. The amendment's text includes the tax parcel numbers of the properties in question: "Subject to the exceptions set forth herein, there shall be only ten MGCE facilities, which shall operate on the following real properties: (1) Being an approximate 40.44 acre area in Butler County, Ohio, identified by the Butler County auditor, as of

February 2, 2015, as tax parcel numbers Q6542084000008 and Q6542084000041"; "Marijuana Reform: Amendment Summary," accessed on August 28, 2015, http://goo.gl/Bm9mVv.

31. Prohibit an Initiated Constitutional Amendment that Would Grant a Monopoly, House Joint Resolution 4, 131st Ohio General Assembly (2015).

32. Matt Pearce, "Ohio Voters Soundly Reject Marijuana Legalization Initiative," *Los Angeles Times*, November 3, 2015, accessed January 11, 2018, http://goo.gl/SQHO1x.

33. "National Drug Threat Assessment Summary," U.S. Department of Justice Drug Enforcement Administration (2014), 25.

34. The DEA has described the shift in cultivation practices toward private lands as an obstacle to law enforcement and eradication; ibid., 26.

35. The downside of this approach is a race to the bottom in which local governments are forced to relax their regulatory standards in order to attract investments.

36. Medical Marijuana, California Assembly Bill No. 243, Chapter 688, California Legislative Information (2015–2016), accessed on October 16, 2017, https://goo.gl/QaSio6. "(a) Pursuant to Section 7 of Article XI of the California Constitution,…a … county may adopt ordinances that establish additional standards, requirements, and regulations for local licenses and permits for commercial cannabis activity."

37. Use and Regulation of Marijuana, Colorado Amendment 64, Section 5(b)(II)(f).

38. This practice was subsequently upheld in *Green Collar LLC v. Pierce County* (2014).

39. Seventy-five cities or counties in Washington have banned marijuana; see "Marijuana Regulation in Washington State," MRSC Local Government Success, accessed on October 16, 2017, http://goo.gl/hBNwfG. As of December 2014, 165 municipalities had banned marijuana in Colorado; see John Aguilar and Jon Murray, "Colorado Cities and Towns Take Diverging Paths on Recreational Pot," *Denver Post*, December 27, 2014, accessed January 11, 2018, http://goo.gl/cVFuyx.

40. "Ordinance No. 01-13, Amending RMC Title 9, Chapters 9.10 & 9.11 Paraphernalia," Council Agenda Coversheet, Richland, Washington City Council, January 15, 2013, accessed on October 16, 2017, http://goo.gl/I2Wn4l.

41. See open letter from Jim Wood, Assemblymember, 2nd District, California Legislature, to California county and city government officials on The Marijuana Regulation and Safety Act's March 1st Deadline (n.d., 2016), http://goo.gl/PH3645.

42. Medical Marijuana: Cultivation Licenses, California Assembly Bill No. 21, Chapter 1, California Legislative Information (2015–2016), accessed on October 16, 2017, https://goo.gl/6QnmNz.

43. See the list of ordinances banning marijuana at "Ban the Bans: Getting Active Locally," California NORML, January 21, 2016, accessed on October 16, 2017, http://www.canorml.org/news/banthebans (spreadsheet, http://goo.gl/bnJL7Z).

44. The final ordinance was substantially based on a model marijuana agriculture ordinance developed by the Cannabis Club Voice Humboldt, and transferred to the Humboldt County Board of Supervisors; see "Humboldt Supervisors to Use CCVH as Framework for Local Marijuana Regulations," News Channel 3, KIEM TV, March 29, 2016; Ryan Burns, "County Takes the Reins on Marijuana Regs as CCVH Steps Back," *Lost Coast Outpost*, September 15, 2015, https://goo.gl/3mkeLU; and interview with Cannabis Club Voice Humboldt by author, Arcata, California, September 10, 2015.

45. Commercial Medical Marijuana Land Use Ordinance, Humboldt County Ordinance No. 2544, 55.4.9 (January 2016).

46. Ibid., 55.4.10.

47. Ibid., 55.4.8.3.

48. Ibid., 55.4.15.

49. Ibid., 55.4.9.

50. Ibid., 55.4.9.4.

51. Ibid., 55.4.14, up to a maximum of 20,000 square feet.

52. Interview with marijuana farmers by author, March 15, 2016.

53. Commercial Medical Marijuana Land Use Ordinance, Humboldt County, Ordinance No. 2544, 55.4.10(e) and 55.4.11(c) (2016).

54. Ibid., 55.4.10. (f), (g), (h), and (i).

55. Ibid., 55.4.11(l). "Where surface water diversion provides any part of the water supply for irrigation of cannabis cultivation, the applicant shall either: 1) consent to forebear from any such diversion during the period from May 15th to October 31st of each year and establish on-site water storage for retention of wet season flows sufficient to provide adequate irrigation water for the size of the area to be cultivated, or 2) submit a water management plan prepared by a qualified person such as a licensed engineer, hydrologist, or similar qualified professional, that establishes minimum water storage and forbearance period, if required, based upon local site conditions, or 3) obtain approval from the RWQCB through enrollment pursuant to NCRWQB Order No.2015-0023 and/or preparation of a Water Resources Protection Plan."

56. Scott Bauer et al., "Impacts of Surface Water Diversion for Marijuana Cultivation on Aquatic Habitat in Four Northwestern California Watersheds," *PLOS One* 10, no. 9 (2015).

57. There are, of course, instances in which water rights must be correlatively curtailed during unusually dry seasons, but I am not aware of any water regulation framework that prohibits water rights holders growing certain crops from making use of their water resources on a seasonal basis.

58. See, e.g., Charles Batchelor et al., "Do Water-Saving Technologies Improve Environmental Flows," *Journal of Hydrology* 518, part A (October 2014): 140, which argues that water-saving methods may often have perverse results on water resources.

59. Commercial Medical Marijuana Land Use Ordinance, Humboldt County, Ordinance No. 2544, 55.4.11(a) (2016).

60. Ibid., 55.4.10.(f), (g), (h), and (i).

61. *Regina v. Parker* (2000), 49 O.R. 3d 481 (Can. Ont. C.A.).

62. Ibid.

63. Ibid.

64. Ibid., ¶10.

65. Ibid., ¶126.

66. Benedict Fischer, Sharan Kuganesan, and Robin Room, "Medical Marijuana Programs: Implications for Cannabis Control Policy—Observations from Canada," *International Journal of Drug Policy* 26 (2015): 15–16.

67. Ibid.

68. Ibid., 16.

69. Philippe G. Lucas, "Regulating Compassion: An Overview of Canada's Federal Medical Cannabis Policy and Practice," *Harm Reduction Journal* 5 (2008): 5.

70. Ibid.

71. *Regina v. J.P.* (2003), 64 O.R. 3d 757, ¶17 (Can. Ont. C.A.).

72. See *Regina v. Long* (2007), 88 O.R. 3d 146, ¶4 (Can. Ont. C.A.).

73. *Sfetkopoulos v. Canada* (2008), FC 33, 399–400 (Can. Ont. Fed. Ct.).

74. "[I]t may well be that there could be justification for limiting the size of operations of designated producers, to facilitate supervision and inspection for quality and security. But any new regulations to this end will have to be justified as having a demonstrable purpose rationally related to legitimate state interests. No such justification has been offered." Ibid., 409.

75. "Canada Medical Marijuana (MMPR) Guide: 25 Questions & Answers," Leaf Science (April 1, 2014), http://www.leafscience.com/2014/04/01/canada-medical-marijuana-mmpr-guide-25-questions-answers/.

76. Ibid.

77. Ibid.

78. "Authorized Licensed Producers of Cannabis for Medical Purposes," Government of Canada, https://www.canada.ca/en/health-canada/services/drugs-health-pro ducts/medical-use-marijuana/licensed-producers/authorized-licensed-producers -medical-purposes.html (last visited July 22, 2017); "Application Process: Becoming a Licensed Producer of Cannabis for Medical Purposes," Government of Canada, https://www.canada.ca/en/health-canada/services/drugs-health-products/medical -use-marijuana/licensed-producers/application-process-becoming-licensed-producer .html (last visited July 22, 2017).

79. *A Framework for the Legalization and Regulation of Cannabis in Canada: The Final Report of the Task Force on Cannabis Legalization and Regulation*, Health Canada (December 2016), http://healthycanadians.gc.ca/task-force-marijuana-groupe-etude /framework-cadre/index-eng.php.

80. Ibid., 4.

81. "An Act Respecting Cannabis and to Amend the Controlled Drugs and Substances Act," House of Commons of Canada, Bill C-45, First Session, Forty-Second Parliament (2017), http://www.parl.ca/DocumentViewer/en/42-1/bill/C-45/first -reading.

82. David Cochrane, "Liberals Want to Move Up Pot Legalization to Avoid Canada Day Celebrations," CBC News, April 8, 2017, http://www.cbc.ca/news/politics/legal -marijuana-date-canada-day-1.4060783.

83. The National Agricultural Law Center compiles an index of publications on these and other topics pertinent to the regulation of agriculture; see "Research Articles," National Agricultural Law Center, accessed on October 16, 2017, http:// goo.gl/qZnRd4.

84. In some cases, the impulse to maintain oversight has prompted states to require vertical integration of the supply chain.

85. *States of Nebraska et al. v. State of Colorado*, Complaint (2014), http://goo.gl /HzKBEZ. The Supreme Court declined to hear the case; see "Orders in Pending Cases," Order List: 577 U.S., Supreme Court, March 21, 2016, accessed October 16, 2017, http://goo.gl/4QJ1Bj.

86. Indoor growing offers many advantages, such as controlled climate, environment, and light. Robert Bergman, *I Love Growing Marijuana: Marijuana Grow Bible*, ebook (2014), https://s3.amazonaws.com/growguides/ILGM-marijuana-grow-bible.pdf.

87. See Ryan Stoa, "Subsidiarity in Principle: Decentralization of Water Resources Management," *Utrecht Law Review* 10, no. 2 (May 2014): 31, https://www.utrecht lawreview.org/articles/abstract/10.18352/ulr.267/.

88. In *Democracy in America*, Alexis de Tocqueville remarked in his comparison of early America with France under Louis XIV that "administrative centralization is suitable only to enervate the peoples who submit to it, because it constantly tends to diminish the spirit of citizenship in them. Administrative centralization, it is true, succeeds in gathering at a given time and in a certain place all the available forces of a nation, but it is harmful to the multiplication of those forces. It brings the nation victory on the day of battle and over time reduces its power. So it can work admirably toward the passing greatness of a man, not toward the lasting prosperity of a people." See Alexis de Tocqueville, *Democracy in America*, vol. 1 (1838; Project Gutenberg, 2006), http://www.gutenberg.org/ebooks/815.

89. Stoa, "Subsidiarity in Principle," 34; see also Graham R. Marshall, "Nesting, Subsidiarity, and Community-Based Environmental Governance beyond the Local Level," *International Journal of the Commons* 2, no. 1 (November 2007): 77, http://doi.org/10.18352/ijc.50; and Elinor Ostrom, "Coping with Tragedies of the Commons," *Annual Review of Political Science* 2, no. 1 (June 1999): 526, https://doi.org/10.1146/annurev.polisci.2.1.493.

90. Galt, California, for example, has banned the indoor or outdoor cultivation of marijuana; see Jennifer Bonnett, "Galt's Medical Marijuana Rule Takes Effect," *Lodi* (CA) *News-Sentinel*, March 5, 2015, http://goo.gl/x8nqxX.

91. Regional Water Quality Control Board, North Coast Region, *Executive Officer's Summary Report* (Santa Rosa, CA: Regional Water Board Office, 2017).

92. "Order R5-2015-0113: Waste Discharge Requirements General Order for Discharges of Waste Associated with Medicinal Cannabis Cultivation Activities," California Regional Water Quality Control Board, Central Valley Region, accessed on October 16, 2017, https://www.waterboards.ca.gov/centralvalley/water_issues/cannabis/general_order/#cannabisgenord.

93. See e.g., "Strategy: Regulation and Enforcement of Unauthorized Diversions; Discharges of Waste to Surface and Groundwater Caused by Marijuana Cultivation," California State Water Resources Control Board (2014).

94. Emily Brady's chronicles of a Humboldt County Deputy Sheriff underline the solitary and seemingly futile efforts to enforce ambiguous marijuana laws in the region. Emily Brady, *Humboldt: Life on America's Marijuana Frontier* (New York: Grand Central Publishing, 2013), 48.

95. See "Annual Update," Colorado Department of Revenue, Enforcement Division—Marijuana (2015).

96. See e.g., "Colorado Department of Agriculture: Factual and Policy Issues Related to the Use of Pesticides on Cannabis" (2016), https://goo.gl/FgFwN2 (noting that the Colorado Department of Agriculture received little guidance from the federal EPA regarding pesticide regulations); and letter from John W. Hickenlooper, Governor of

Colorado, to Tom Vilsack, Secretary of the U.S. Department of Agriculture, February 20, 2014, https://goo.gl/jQn4iD, requesting assistance from the federal Department of Agriculture on industrial hemp cultivation.

97. "Colorado Department of Agriculture: Factual and Policy Issues."

98. To take a broader view of this point, cooperative federalism frameworks between the federal and state governments (such as the regulatory structures for the Clean Water Act or Clean Air Act) have been effective because they utilize the federal government's funding streams and establish minimum standards to support state-level programs, which then remain relatively coherent from a national perspective; see e.g., Robert L. Fischman, "Cooperative Federalism and Natural Resources Law," *New York University Environmental Law Journal* 14 (2005): 179; Douglas Williams, "Toward Regional Governance in Environmental Law," *Akron Law Review* 46, no. 4 (2013); and Ryan B. Stoa, "Cooperative Federalism in Biscayne National Park," *Natural Resources Journal* 56, no. 1 (2016): 81.

99. See also Ryan B. Stoa, "Water Governance in Haiti: An Assessment of Laws and Institutional Capacities," *Tulane Environmental Law Journal* 29, no. 2 (2017): 243.

100. Editorial Board, "The Challenge of 'Big Marijuana,'" The Monitor's View, *Christian Science Monitor*, March 7, 2016, https://www.csmonitor.com/Commentary/the-monitors-view/2016/0307/The-challenge-of-Big-Marijuana.

101. California Proposition 64 (California Adult Use of Marijuana Act of 2016), §26061(d).

102. *The State of Legal Marijuana Markets*, 5th ed. (Arcview Market Research, 2017).

103. *Cultivation: Capitalizing on a Tripling of Legal Demand*, Cannabis Intelligence Briefing, 5th ed. (Arcview Market Research, 2017).

104. Sungnome Madrone, interview with the author, May 22, 2017.

105. "2016 Final Domestic Cannabis Eradication/Suppression Program Statistical Report," United States Drug Enforcement Administration (2016), https://www.dea.gov/ops/cannabis_2016.pdf.

106. Sungnome Madrone, interview with the author, May 22, 2017.

Chapter 5

1. California Cannabis Voice Humboldt, for example, is a grassroots organization that works "to preserve the ideals of the small family cannabis farm."

2. Some scholars believe *Cannabis ruderalis* to be a third species of the *Cannabis* genus. Others believe it is a subspecies of *Cannabis sativa*.

3. One such list, compiled by Leafly.com, counts 779 well-established strains.

4. See Jason Sawler et al., "The Genetic Structure of Marijuana and Hemp," *PLOS One* 10, no. 8 (August 2015): 1371, https://doi.org/10.1371/journal.pone.0133292.

5. Michael Pollan, *The Botany of Desire* (New York: Random House, 2001), 132.

6. The actual name of the strain has been changed.

7. Karl Marx, "A Contribution to the Critique of Political Economy," in *Marx and Engels Collected Works*, vol. 29, trans. S. W. Ryazanskaya (Moscow: Progress Publishers, 1986), first published online at Marx.org (1993); reprinted, Marxists.org (1999), https://goo.gl/cK2kOw.

8. "'Agricultural Commodity' Defined," Title 7 U.S. Code §1518 (1938).

9. "Commoditize," Investopedia, accessed October 2, 2017, http://goo.gl/u4hJVN.

10. Martin Rapaport, "Commoditization: Diamond Industry to Establish Fair, Open, Competitive Markets," *Rapaport Magazine*, July 1, 2007.

11. See "Egg Farm Price Received Data," YCharts, accessed March 28, 2016, https://goo.gl/yEqjo4.

12. See Dan Charles, "Most U.S. Egg Producers Are Now Choosing Cage-Free Houses," *The Salt*, National Public Radio, January 15, 2016, http://goo.gl/bqWAUf.

13. See Shruti Date Singh and Lydia Mulvany, "Egg Markets Disrupted in the U.S. as Cages Made Roomier," *Bloomberg Business*, December 12, 2014, http://goo.gl/5fUQS3.

14. See, e.g., "Appellations of origin," 27 Code of Federal Regulations (C.F.R.) §4.25 (2001).

15. The *Economist*'s February 13, 2016, cover story on marijuana regulation finds the emergence of large-scale agricultural companies and consolidation of the industry likely. "Legalising Cannabis: Reeferegulatory Challenge," *Economist*, February 13, 2016, http://goo.gl/UggQeM.

16. Tom Capehart, "Trends in U.S. Tobacco Farming," *USDA: Electronic Research Service*, November 2004.

17. Ross Hammond, "Consolidation in the Tobacco Industry," *Tobacco Control* 7, no. 4 (December 1998): 426.

18. See, e.g., John Maxfield, "The Making of Colorado's Marijuana Millionaires," *The Motley Fool*, January 4, 2014, http://goo.gl/uzOW3C; John Ingold, "Colorado Medical-Marijuana Businesses Have Declined by 40 Percent," *Denver Post*, March 2, 2013, http://goo.gl/gThz7W.

19. Trademark registration requires lawful use of the mark in commerce, and Section 2(a) of the Lanham Act bars registration for an "immoral, deceptive, or

scandalous matter." The U.S. Patent and Trademark Office (USPTO) has declared that because marijuana is illegal under federal law, marijuana strains would constitute an immoral or scandalous matter.

20. Hilary Bricken, "The Possibility of Marijuana Plant Patents," *Above the Law,* July 6, 2015, accessed January 12, 2018, http://goo.gl/DIitUP.

21. Greg Walters, "What a Looming Patent War Could Mean for the Future of the Marijuana Industry," *Vice,* April 20, 2016, https://news.vice.com/article/a-patent-for-cannabis-plants-is-already-a-reality-and-more-are-expected-to-follow.

22. Julie Weed, "US Patent Office Issuing Cannabis Patents to a Growing Market," *Forbes,* July 24, 2017, accessed January 12, 2018, https://www.forbes.com/sites/julieweed/2017/07/24/us-patent-office-issuing-cannabis-patents-to-a-growing-market/#479fbab568d4.

23. See also Jonathan Caulkins's study, *Results from the 2013 National Survey on Drug Use and Health: Summary of National Findings,* Substance Abuse and Mental Health Services Administration (Rockville, MD, 2014), 26.

24. Jonathan Caulkins et al., *Considering Marijuana Legalization: Insights for Vermont and Other Jurisdictions* (Santa Monica, CA: RAND Corporation, 2015), 139–140.

25. Jonathan P. Caulkins, *Marijuana Legalization: What Everyone Needs to Know,* 2nd ed. (New York: Oxford University Press, 2016).

26. *The State of Legal Marijuana Markets,* 5th ed. (Arcview Market Research, 2017), 71.

27. With the fall in prices, some farmers have dropped their rate to $150 per pound.

28. Jeffrey Michael, director of the Center for Business and Policy Research, University of the Pacific, in an interview with the author, June 2017.

29. Quoted in Walters, "What a Looming Patent War Could Mean."

30. "U.S. Beer Sales Volume Growth 2016," National Beer Sales & Production Data, *Brewers Association,* accessed March 26, 2018, https://www.brewersassociation.org/statistics/national-beer-sales-production-data/.

31. Daniel G. Barrus et al., "Tasty THC: Promises and Challenges of Cannabis Edibles," *Methods Report* (RTI Press, 2016), 10.3768/rtipress.2016.op.0035.1611.

32. *The State of Legal Marijuana Markets,* 68.

33. And if that's the case, maybe production costs of $8 to $33 per pound really are possible.

34. Bailey Rahn, "Terpenes: The Flavors of Cannabis Aromatherapy," Leafly.com, February 12, 2014, accessed January 12, 2018, https://www.leafly.com/news/cannabis-101/terpenes-the-flavors-of-cannabis-aromatherapy.

35. *The State of Legal Marijuana Markets*, 71.

36. Pre-rolled products consist of crumbled buds that have been rolled into a paper, ready to be smoked.

37. "Plant vs. Utility Patents," Perennial Patent Company, accessed October 3, 2017, http://perennialpatents.com/plantpatent-v-utility-patents/.

38. "Utility Patents," Perennial Patent Company, accessed October 3, 2017, http://www.bios.net/daisy/bios/1234#utility_patents.

39. Amanda Chicago Lewis, "The Great Pot Monopoly Mystery," *GQ*, August 23, 2017, https://www.gq.com/story/the-great-pot-monopoly-mystery.

40. Winston Ross, "The Man Mapping the Marijuana Genome Is Changing the Weed Game," *Newsweek*, March 14, 2016, accessed January 12, 2018, http://www.newsweek.com/2016/03/25/marijuana-scientist-mapping-cannabis-genome-changing-weed-game-436526.html.

41. A clone planted too early in the spring might be confused by the lack of daylight and think autumn has arrived, triggering the plant's flowering phase four to five months early.

42. "Senescence," *Nature*, accessed October 3, 2017, https://www.nature.com/subjects/senescence.

43. Another way of looking at it is that the farmer is cultivating a single plant year after year. After ten years, the plant is still alive by means of cloning, but the plant is ten years old all the same.

44. Seeded plants will always have a place in the marijuana industry because they are necessary to keep the industry moving forward as well. Clones represent a replica of a plant or strain already in existence. In order to create a new hybrid, two plants must reproduce together and create seeds. Take, for example, the ongoing arms race to produce the world's most THC-potent marijuana. The record, as of 2017, is around 34 percent THC. A clone taken from that plant will produce buds that also contain 34 percent THC. But if a breeder wants to break that record, clones will never help because they will always contain 34 percent THC. Breeding two plants together may produce 9,999 plants that come nowhere close to breaking the record. But it's possible that seeded plant number 10,000 will break the record, and that possibility is what allows seeded plants to keep the industry moving forward.

45. Some males might be kept in order to harvest their pollen and stimulate reproduction.

46. Technically, all marijuana plants can "hermaph," or become hermaphrodites. In these relatively rare cases, the plant develops both male and female flowers.

47. A. C. Noé, "Gottlieb Haberlandt," *Plant Physiology* 9 (1934): 851–855.

48. Roberta H. Smith, *Plant Tissue Culture: Techniques and Experiments*, 3rd ed. (London: Elsevier, 2013), 1; Ian M. Sussex, "The Scientific Roots of Modern Plant Technology," *Plant Cell* 20, no. 5 (May 2008): 1189, https://www.ncbi.nlm.nih.gov /pmc/articles/PMC2438469/; and Trevor Thorpe, "History of Plant Cell Culture," in *Plant Tissue Culture: Techniques and Experiments*, 3rd ed. (London: Elsevier, 2013), 2.

Chapter 6

1. Extract from Thomas Jefferson's letter to Jean Guillaume Hyde de Neuville, December 13, 1818, Monticello.org, accessed October 17, 2017, http://tjrs.monticello.org /letter/364.

2. "Cabot Vineyard 2007 Cabernet Sauvignon (Humboldt County)," Wine and Ratings, *Wine Enthusiast*, accessed October 4, 2017, http://www.winemag.com/buying -guide/cabot-vineyards-2007-cabernet-sauvignon-humboldt-county/.

3. "Bubba Kush," Strain Highlights, Leafly.com, accessed October 4, 2017, https:// www.leafly.com/indica/bubba-kush.

4. David White, *But First, Champagne* (New York: Skyhorse Publishing, 2016).

5. Mike Veseth, *Money, Taste, and Wine: It's Complicated!* (Lanham, MD: Rowman & Littlefield, 2015), 114.

6. Related terms include "designation of origin" or "geographical indication."

7. In the wine industry, for example, the appellation system in the United States is only concerned with geography, while the European Union's appellations typically require more stringent standards be met.

8. See Michael Maher, "On Vino Veritas? Clarifying the Use of Geographic References on American Wine Labels," *California Law Review* 89, no. 6 (December 2001): 1884.

9. See Jancis Robinson, *Oxford Companion to Wine*, 3rd ed. (Oxford, UK: Oxford University Press, 1994), 322.

10. Appellations of Origin, 27 Code of Federal Regulations (C.F.R.) §4.25 (2012).

11. See e.g., "Wine Appellations of Origin," U.S. Department of the Treasury, Alcohol and Tobacco Tax and Trade Bureau, accessed October 5, 2017, https://www.ttb .gov/appellation/index.shtml. The TTB website states that for states and counties, not less than 75 percent of the volume of the wine must be derived from grapes grown in the labeled appellation, and in AVAs, not less than 85 percent.

12. See Alyson M. Chouinard, "Wine Appellation Regulation in the U.S. and France as a Response to Globalization," *Inquiries Journal* 3, no. 1 (2011), http://goo.gl/fVWlg3.

13. Of course, the model also fosters fraud, as lesser or outside cultivators attempt to claim a region as their own or simply confuse the consumer. See Jay Kiiha, "Trade

Protectionism of Wine Brand Names at the Expense of American Viticultural Areas: Arbitrary Protection of 'Big Liquor' at the Expense of Small Vineyards," *Drake Journal of Agricultural Law* 9, no. 1 (Spring 2004): 159.

14. See Mike Veseth, "How Champagne Changed the Global Economy," *Fortune Magazine*, August 4, 2015, https://perma.cc/AZJ2-C4GT. Veseth writes: "The appellation system was a defensive mechanism, meant to ward off foreign foes and domestic saboteurs, and it is perhaps not surprising how quickly the idea spread at a time when economic threats were seemingly numberless and promises of security particularly precious."

15. The European Union's agricultural product quality scheme states: "Assisting producers, by means of the operation of quality schemes, to be rewarded for their efforts to produce a diversity of quality products, can benefit the rural economy. This is particularly the case in less favored areas, where the farming sector accounts for a significant part of the economy. In this way quality schemes contribute to and complement rural development policy as well as market and income support policies." European Commission, "Proposal for a Regulation of the European Parliament and of the Council on Agricultural Product Quality Schemes" (Brussels, 2010).

16. Ibid.

17. See Veseth, *Money, Taste, and Wine*, for a description of the rise of counterfeit champagne production in the absence of legitimate producers.

18. The French appellation responsible for regulating the production of Comté cheese, for example, has "used the production specifications to reduce concentration (of the fruitières and the farms), to maintain the quality of the cheese, and to preserve the traditional production methods." See Amy B. Trubek and Sarah Bowen, "Creating the Taste of Place in the United States: Can We Learn from the French?," *GeoJournal* 73, no. 1 (2008): 26.

19. Maher, "On Vino Veritas?," 1885–1886.

20. See Elizabeth Barham, "Translating Terroir: The Global Challenge of French AOC Labeling," *Journal of Rural Studies* 19, no. 1 (2003): 133, https://doi.org/10.1016/S0743-0167(02)00052-9.

21. See ibid., 134–135.

22. European Commission, "Quality Schemes."

23. My father was raised in rural Minnesota by Midwestern parents who lived through the Great Depression and recognized the value of preserving scarce resources.

24. Andrew Jefford, "Jefford on Monday: Burgundy's Other Self," *Decanter*, June 5, 2017, http://www.decanter.com/wine-news/opinion/jefford-on-monday/cremant-de-bourgogne-wine-guide-370176/.

25. Tony Dokoupil, "Vice Wars: Tobacco, Alcohol and the Rise of Big Marijuana," NBC News, November 29, 2014, accessed January 11, 2018, http://goo.gl/CrXqSB.

26. John Bershaw et al., "Cannabis Terroir: Where Is the Grass Greener?," *Geological Society of America* 49, no. 6 (2017).

27. While there are myriad problems with the Jamaican marijuana industry and little research on the subject, there is anecdotal evidence that indigenous strains are well adapted and can produce quality marijuana. See Pete Brady, "Ganja Gardens," *Cannabis Culture*, October 25, 2002, http://goo.gl/6Cioxi.

28. See e.g., "Outdoor Cannabis Seeds," Sensi Seeds, accessed October 6, 2017, https://goo.gl/PKEoh4; "Cannabis Seeds for Cool Climate," Barney's Farm Seeds, accessed October 6, 2017, https://goo.gl/benIZk.

29. "Main Grape Varieties by European Wine Region," 1885 Consulting, accessed October 6, 2017, http://goo.gl/zNiZPh.

30. Which, over time, effectively becomes a brand.

31. Toby Keith, "Wacky Tobaccy," track 2 on *The Bus Songs*, Show Dog-Universal Music, 2017.

32. 311, "Nutsymptom," track 3 on *Grassroots*, Capricorn, 1993.

33. Z-Ro, "1st Time Again," featuring Ashanti, track 12 on *Let the Truth Be Told*, Asylum, Rap-A-Lot, 2005.

34. Redman, "Blow Treez," featuring Ready Roc and Method Man, track 13 on *Red Gone Wild: Thee Album*, 2007.

35. Nas, "World's an Addiction," featuring Anthony Hamilton, track 7 on *Life Is Good*, 2012.

36. Big KRIT, "Mind Control," featuring Wiz Khalifa and E-40, track 8 on *Cadillactica*, 2014.

37. Wiz Khalifa, "KK," featuring Juicy J and Project Pat, track 4 on *Blacc Hollywood*, 2014.

38. Master P, "1/2 on a Bag of Dank," track 4 on *Ice Cream Man*, 1996.

39. *The State of Legal Marijuana Markets*, 5th ed. (Arcview Market Research, 2017), 69.

40. See e.g., Jon Gettman, "Lost Taxes and Other Costs of Marijuana Laws," Drug Science (2007), accessed on October 6, 2017, http://goo.gl/pVfTrz. Beau Kilmer, co-director of the Drug Policy Research Center, estimates that two-thirds of the marijuana consumed in the United States in 2008 was sourced in Mexico; cited in Deborah Bonello, "Mexican Marijuana Farmers See Profits Tumble as U.S. Loosens

Laws," *Los Angeles Times*, December 30, 2015, accessed January 11, 2018, http://goo.gl/udEjtG. Other estimates complicate the picture, claiming that by 2010, 80 percent of marijuana consumed in the United States came from California. See Emily Brady, "How Humboldt Became America's Marijuana Capital," *Salon*, June 30, 2013, http://goo.gl/529p1p.

41. See, e.g., William Neuman, "As Drug Kingpins Fall in Mexico, Cartels Fracture and Violence Surges," *New York Times*, August 12, 2015, http://goo.gl/sJTBzC.

42. Bonello, "Mexican Marijuana Farmers See Profits Tumble as U.S. Loosens Laws."

43. Appellations, 27 C.F.R. §4.25 (2012).

44. In *Bronco Wine Co. v. Jolly* (2004), a more restrictive state wine labeling statute was not preempted by federal regulations, for example.

45. See Laura Zanzig, "The Perfect Pairing: Protecting U.S. Geographical Indicators with a Sino-American Wine Registry," *Washington Law Review* 88 (2013): 724.

46. For example, California Cannabis Voice Humboldt and Emerald Growers Association represent marijuana farmers in northern California. See "Who Is California Cannabis Voice Humboldt (CCVH)?," California Cannabis Voice Humboldt, https://perma.cc/PX26-3U7J; "Emerald Growers Association," MedicalJane, accessed October 6, 2017, https://www.medicaljane.com/directory/company/emerald-growers-association/.

47. See Appellations, 27 C.F.R. §4.25(e)(1) (2012).

48. See 27 C.F.R. §9.21–218 (2012).

49. See Tim Unwin, *Wine and the Vine: An Historical Geography of Viticulture and the Wine Trade* (New York: Routledge, 1991), 29.

50. It isn't a given that strict labeling standards are beneficial; in some cases strict requirements may frustrate efforts to adapt to changes in consumer preferences. Old World winemakers have struggled to adapt to the wine market's increasing interest in wines that market a grape varietal instead of a region, for example.

51. See Erica Freeman, "Demand for Organic Cannabis Growing, Too," *Coloradoan*, May 5, 2016, accessed October 6, 2017, http://goo.gl/wauJUr.

52. See Donna Jones, "Organic Marijuana Can't Exist, Which Troubles Growers," *Los Angeles Times*, August 20, 2011, accessed October 6, 2017, http://goo.gl/VSFLBt.

53. The potential of using appellations to regulate environmental impacts and sustainable cultivation methods is discussed at length in chapter 8.

54. Medical Marijuana Regulation and Safety Act, California State S.B. 643 (2015). See also "Assembly Members Urge Governor Brown to Sign Medical Marijuana

Package," News Channel 3, KIEM TV, accessed October 6, 2017, https://perma.cc /K4D7-WY6L, which quotes Jim Wood, 2nd Assembly District, as stating that "cultivators are going to have to comply with the same kinds of regulations that typical farmers do. ... [I]t's going to be treated like an agriculture product."

55. Compassionate Use Act, California Health and Safety Code §11362.5 (2017) accessed on October 6, 2017, https://leginfo.legislature.ca.gov/faces/codes_display-Section.xhtml?lawCode=HSC&sectionNum=11362.5.

56. Medical Marijuana, S.B. 643 §§19332(a)–(e) (2015).

57. Ibid., §19332.5(b).

58. Ibid., §19332.5(d).

59. As of 2015, California had approximately 50,000 marijuana farms accounting for 60 percent of all marijuana grown in the United States. See Alissa Walker, "How Growing More Weed Can Help California Fix Its Water Problems," *Gizmodo*, October 12, 2015, accessed October 6, 2017, http://goo.gl/ZEwFpT.

60. See Cynthia Sweeney, "Mendocino County Divided into Cannabis Appellations," *North Bay Business Journal*, June 13, 2016, accessed October 6, 2017, http://goo .gl/fBgoWC; Keith Mansur, "Cannabis Appellation Regions for Oregon: A Solution for Unwanted Cross-Pollination of Hemp and Marijuana," *Oregon Cannabis Connection*, July 22, 2016, accessed January 12, 2018, https://olis.leg.state.or.us/liz/2015R1 /Downloads/CommitteeMeetingDocument/78941.

61. Sweeney, "Mendocino County Divided into Cannabis Appellations."

62. Ibid.

63. One wine appellation expert, remarking on Justin's approach, noted, "I like the way he's gone about it, because he's factored in not just the natural elements; he's gone out and spoken to growers, asking the old-timers what they think, and is making revisions. He's being true to the history. This is a template for the future, creating a dossier of physical and human, historical factors—I applaud him for that." See http://www.northbaybusinessjournal.com/northbay/mendocinocounty /5702907-181/mendocino-cannabis-appellations.

64. As noted earlier, the agency has the authority to create marijuana appellations pursuant to amendment of the Compassionate Use Act, California Health and Safety Act, California Statute 719 §19332.5(b) (2015).

65. Ryan Reaves, "Envisioning California Cannabis Appellations," *CannaBusiness Law*, August 25, 2017, accessed October 6, 2017, http://cannabusinesslaw.com/2017 /08/envisioning-california-cannabis-appellations/.

66. "Humboldt Proof of Origin," County of Humboldt, accessed October 6, 2017, https://www.humboldtorigin.org/project.xhtml.

67. Resolution Relating to the Regulation of Storefront-Based Medical Cannabis Dispensaries, Humboldt County, Ordinance No. 2544, Resolution No. 16-85 55.4.9 (July 19, 2016).

68. Ibid., 55.4.15.

69. See Mansur, "Cannabis Appellation Regions for Oregon."

70. Quoted in "Vice Wars: Tobacco, Alcohol and the Rise of Big Marijuana," *NBC News*, November 29, 2014, accessed October 6, 2017, https://www.nbcnews.com /storyline/legal-pot/vice-wars-tobacco-alcohol-rise-big-marijuana-n253801.

71. Kolleen M. Guy, *When Champagne Became French* (Baltimore: Johns Hopkins University Press, 2003).

Chapter 7

1. "American Presidents on the Importance of Agriculture," Farm Policy Facts (website), accessed October 17, 2017, https://www.farmpolicyfacts.org/2016/02/american -presidents-on-the-importance-of-agriculture/.

2. Ryan Stoa, "Is Big Marijuana Inevitable? Regulating Marijuana Like Wine Could Prevent Monopolies Post-Legalization," *New Republic*, August 19, 2016, https:// newrepublic.com/article/136172/big-marijuana-inevitable.

3. C. Suetonius Tranquillus, *The Lives of the Twelve Caesars: The Life of Tiberius* (Boston: Loeb Classical Library, 1913), 291, accessed January 12, 2018, http://penel ope.uchicago.edu/Thayer/E/Roman/Texts/Suetonius/12Caesars/Tiberius*.html#37.

4. Jules Janick, Harry S. Paris, and David C. Parrish, "The Cucurbits of Mediterranean Antiquity: Identification of Taxa from Ancient Images and Descriptions," *Annals of Botany* 100, no. 7 (December 2007): 1457, 10.1093/aob/mcm242.

5. "The Orangery," Château de Versailles (website), accessed October 8, 2017, http:// en.chateauversailles.fr/discover/estate/gardens/orangery#the-building.

6. Gwen Bruno, "A Short History of the Greenhouse," Dave's Garden (website), March 1, 2012, accessed October 8, 2017, https://davesgarden.com/guides/articles /view/3607.

7. Ibid.

8. S. H. Wittwer and Wm. Robb, "Carbon Dioxide Enrichment of Greenhouse Atmospheres for Food Crop Production," *Economic Botany* 18, no. 1 (January 1964); Roger H. Thayer, "Carbon Dioxide Enrichment Methods," Hydrofarm.com, accessed on October 10, 2017, https://www.hydrofarm.com/resources/articles/co2_enrich ment.php.

9. Industrial development presented mutual benefits in this regard; many commercial greenhouses partner with industrial facilities to capture the CO_2 waste produced by the facility and release it into the greenhouse.

10. Frank Viviano, "This Tiny Country Feeds the World," *National Geographic*, September 2017, http://www.nationalgeographic.com/magazine/2017/09/holland -agriculture-sustainable-farming/.

11. Ibid.

12. "Quick Facts and Figures about the Dutch Horticultural Industry," Holland, Rijksoverheid (website), accessed October 8, 2017, https://www.hollandtradeandinvest .com/key-sectors/horticulture-and-starting-materials/horticulture-facts-and-figures.

13. Merle H. Jensen and Alan Malter, "Protected Agriculture: A Global Review," World Bank Technical Paper Number 253 (International Bank for Reconstruction and Development, Washington, DC, 1995), 103.

14. United Nations, Department of Economics and Social Affairs, Population Division, "World Population Prospects: Key Findings and Advance Tables, 2017 Revision," Working Paper No. ESA/P/WP/248 (2017), 1, https://esa.un.org/unpd/wpp/Publica tions/Files/WPP2017_KeyFindings.pdf.

15. Food and Agriculture Organization of the United Nations, *The State of Food Security and Nutrition in the World 2017: Building Resilience for Peace and Food Security* (Rome: FAO 2017), http://www.fao.org/state-of-food-security-nutrition/en/.

16. "Farming: Habitat Conversion & Loss," World Wide Fund for Nature, accessed October 8, 2017, http://wwf.panda.org/what_we_do/footprint/agriculture/impacts /habitat_loss/; "Farming: Wasteful Water Use," World Wide Fund for Nature, wwf .panda.org, accessed on October 8, 2017, http://wwf.panda.org/what_we_do/foot print/agriculture/impacts/water_use/.

17. Nikos Alexsandratos and Jelle Bruinsma, Global Perspective and Studies Team, "World Agriculture towards 2030/2050," ESA Working Paper 12-03 (Agricultural Development Economics Division, Food and Agriculture Organization of the United Nations, June 2012), http://www.fao.org/docrep/016/ap106e/ap106e.pdf.

18. Ibid., 13.

19. Ibid., 14.

20. To be fair, concerns about food supplies and the human population have preoccupied scholars for centuries. Thomas Malthus's 1798 book *An Essay on the Principle of Population* is perhaps the most well-known example. Malthus believed that because the human population grows exponentially while food production grows arithmetically, a catastrophic population collapse will inevitably result from a global food shortage. Critics of Malthus point to advances in family planning and

agricultural productivity as proof that the theory is incorrect. Yet proponents argue that the basic idea is still valid: the human population is growing at an alarming rate, and may eventually outstrip available resources.

21. "Factory Fresh," Technology Quarterly: The Future of Agriculture, *Economist* (June 9, 2016), accessed October 8, 2017, http://www.economist.com/technology -quarterly/2016-06-09/factory-fresh.

22. Ian Frazier, "The Vertical Farm: Growing Crops in the City, without Soil or Natural Light," *New Yorker*, January 9, 2017, https://www.newyorker.com/magazine /2017/01/09/the-vertical-farm.

23. Jeff Read, "Why Chicago Is Becoming the Country's Urban Farming Capital," World Changing Ideas, *Fast Company*, June 3, 2016, https://www.fastcompany.com /3059721/why-chicago-is-becoming-the-countrys-urban-farming-capital.

24. "Vertical Farming Market Growing at 30.7% CAGR to 2020 Dominated by Lighting and Hydroponic Components," *ReportsnReports*, January 19, 2016, http:// www.prnewswire.com/news-releases/vertical-farming-market-growing-at-307-cagr -to-2020-dominated-by-lighting--hydroponic-components-565731651.html.

25. Alyssa Bereznak, "Buying the Farm," *Ringer*, April 11, 2017, https://www.theringer .com/2017/4/11/16041798/urban-farming-tech-silicon-valley-f3bb7434c4f0.

26. Laura Riley, "For Farmer Dave and Indoor Farming, Things Are Looking Up," *Tampa Bay Times*, December 2, 2015, http://www.tampabay.com/things-to-do/con sumer/for-farmer-dave-and-indoor-farming-things-are-looking-up/2256055.

27. Sativa strains, as explained in chapter 5, tend to be tall, skinny, and slow to flower.

28. *Cannabis Intelligence Briefing*, 5th ed. (Arcview Market Research, 2017), 24.

29. "Electric Power Monthly: With Data for January 2018," Independent Statistics and Analysis, U.S. Energy Information Administration, U.S. Department of Energy (March 2018), https://www.eia.gov/electricity/monthly/epm_table_grapher.php ?t=epmt_5_6_a.

30. *Cannabis Intelligence Briefing*, 19.

Chapter 8

1. Kelsey Burton, "What Did Past Presidents Have to Say about Agriculture?," *VA-Leaders-OR: Leadership for Virginia's Largest Industry* (blog), February 18, 2013.

2. Upton Sinclair, *The Jungle* (Mineola, NY: Dover Publications, 2001).

3. James M. Cole, Deputy Attorney General, U.S. Department of Justice, "Memorandum for All United States Attorneys: Guidance Regarding Marijuana Enforcement," August 29, 2013, https://www.justice.gov/iso/opa/resources/3052013829132756857467.pdf.

4. Office of Governor Edmund G. Brown, Jr., "Governor Brown Declares Drought State of Emergency," ca.gov, January 17, 2014, http://gov.ca.gov/news.php ?id=18368.

5. Ibid.

6. Josh Harkinson, "The Landscape-Scarring, Energy-Sucking, Wildlife-Killing Reality of Pot Farming: This Is Your Wilderness on Drugs," *Mother Jones*, March/April 2014, http://www.motherjones.com/environment/2014/03/marijuana-weed-pot-farming -environmental-impacts/.

7. Scott Bauer et al., "Impacts of Surface Water Diversion for Marijuana Cultivation on Aquatic Habitat in Four Northwestern California Watersheds," *PLOS One* 10, no. 9 (March 18, 2015), https://doi.org/10.1371/journal.pone.0120016.

8. Andrew Goff, "Major Multi-Agency Marijuana Raid in Island Mountain Today," *Lost Coast Outpost*, June 22, 2015, http://lostcoastoutpost.com/2015/jun/22/major -marijuana-raid-island-mountain-today/.

9. Nancy Capace, *The Encyclopedia of California*, 8th ed. (St. Clair Shores, MI: Somer-set Publishers, 1999), 285.

10. Adam Randall, "Tri-County Pot Raids Net 86,578 Plants," *Chico Enterprise-Record*, June 29, 2015, http://www.chicoer.com/general-news/20150629/tri-county-pot -raids-net-86578-plants.

11. Ibid.

12. Goff, "Major Multi-Agency Marijuana Raid."

13. Randall, "Operation 'Emerald Tri-County' Nets 86,578 Marijuana Plants."

14. Ibid.

15. Ryan Burns, "Yesterday's Pot Bust Involved Members of California Cannabis Voice Humboldt," *Lost Coast Outpost*, June 23, 2015, http://lostcoastoutpost.com /2015/jun/23/yesterdays-pot-bust-involved-members-california-ca/; Josh Harkinson, "Police Say the Biggest Pot Raid in Years Wasn't Really about Pot: Forget the Drug War—The Main Battle Now in the Emerald Triangle May Be Drought," *Mother Jones*, June 30, 2015, http://www.motherjones.com/environment/2015/06/emerald -triangle-marijuana-raid-water-drought.

16. Burns, "Yesterday's Pot Bust."

17. One researcher at the Humboldt Institute for Interdisciplinary Marijuana Research described the delicate political situation surrounding marijuana research succinctly: "At my university, there is nobody who will even go near it." Harkinson, "The Landscape-Scarring, Energy-Sucking, Wildlife-Killing Reality of Pot Farming."

18. Compassionate Care Act, New York State Assembly: A06357 (2014), accessed on October 9, 2017, http://goo.gl/4fXESQ; see also Jesse McKinley, "New York State Awards 5 Million Medical Marijuana Licenses, *New York Times*, July 21, 2015, http://goo.gl/3b3iwl.

19. The bill's summary begins, "Relates to the medical use of marihuana; legalizes the possession, manufacture, use, delivery, transport or administration of medical marihuana by a designated caregiver for a certified medical use."

20. "Manufacturing of medical marihuana by a registered organization shall only be done in an indoor, enclosed, secure facility located in New York State, which may include a greenhouse." Compassionate Care Act, New York State Assembly: A06357 (2014).

21. Task Force Report on the Implementation of Prop 64, "Regulation of Marijuana in Colorado" (Office of the Governor, 2013), https://www.colorado.gov/pacific/sites /default/files/A64TaskForceFinalReport%5B1%5D_1.pdf; Bryce Pardo, "Cannabis Policy Reforms in the Americas: A Comparative Analysis of Colorado, Washington, and Uruguay," *International Journal of Drug Policy* 25, no. 4 (July 2014): 727, https:// doi.org/10.1016/j.drugpo.2014.05.010; see Taxes on Marijuana and Marijuana Products, Colorado Session 69 H.B. 1318 (2017). The task force's recommendations were largely adopted by the state legislature and passed in May 2013. See Retail Marijuana, Colorado Session 69 H.B. 13-1317 (2013); Amendment 64 Appropriation, Colorado Session S.B. 283 (2013).

22. David Migoya, "Colorado Yields to Marijuana Industry Pressure on Pesticides," Business, *Denver Post*, October 3, 2015, http://www.denverpost.com/2015/10/03 /colorado-yields-to-marijuana-industry-pressure-on-pesticides/.

23. See Ryan Stoa, "Weed and Water Law: Regulating Legal Marijuana," *Hastings Law Journal* 67, no. 3 (2016).

24. "Bureau of Reclamation—About Us—Fact Sheet," Reclamation: Managing Water in the West, U.S. Bureau of Reclamation, last updated November 22, 2017, http:// www.usbr.gov/main/about/fact.html.

25. Ibid.

26. "Reclamation Manual: Temporary Release (Expires 5/16/2018)," Reclamation: Managing Water in the West, U.S. Bureau of Reclamation, accessed on October 9, 2017, http://www.usbr.gov/recman/temporary_releases/pectrmr-63.pdf.

27. "Bureau of Reclamation—About Us."

28. Rob Hotakainen, "With No Federal Water, Pot Growers Could Be High and Dry," *McClatchy Washington Bureau*, April 27, 2014, http://www.mcclatchydc.com /news/nation-world/national/article24766780.html.

29. Ibid.

30. Nicholas K. Geranios and Gene Johnson, "Feds Don't Want Irrigation Water Used to Grow Pot," Associated Press, *Denver Post*, May 20, 2014, http://www.denverpost .com/marijuana/ci_25799421/.

31. Matt Ferner and Mollie Reilly, "Feds May Cut Off Water for Legal Marijuana Crops," Politics, *Huffington Post*, May 19, 2014, http://goo.gl/oCO0UH.

32. Ibid.

33. See, e.g., Marijuana Water Regulations, St. Charles Mesa Water District: Regulations §5.08, accessed on October 9, 2017, http://www.stcharlesmesawaterdistrict.org /index.php/20-regulations/153-marijuana-water-regulations.

34. Stoa, "Weed and Water Law 30, 56 (text accompanying Riparianism).

35. Ibid., 56.

36. Ibid., 57; see also Charles J. P. Podolak and Martin Doyle, "Conditional Water Rights in the Western United States: Introducing Uncertainty to Prior Appropriation?" *Journal of the American Water Resources Association* 15, no. 14 (2014), 10.1111/ jawr.12229.

37. Ibid., 57.

38. Medical Marijuana Regulation and Safety Act [MMRSA], California Statute AB 243 (2015); California Statute AB 266 (2015); Cal Statute SB 643 (2015).

39. MMRSA California Statute AB 243 §§19332(a)–(e).

40. Craig Thompson et al., "Impacts of Rodenticide and Insecticide Toxicants from Marijuana Cultivation Sites on Fisher Survival Rates in the Sierra National Forest, California," *Conservation Letters* 7, no. 2 (2014): 91.

41. Jennifer K. Carah et al., "High Time for Conservation: Adding the Environment to the Debate on Marijuana Liberalization," *BioScience* 65, no. 8 (June 2015): 3–4, https://doi.org/10.1093/biosci/biv083, citing Jim F. Milestone et al., "Continued Cultivation of Illegal Marijuana in U.S. Western National Parks, Proceedings from the 2011 George Wright Society Conference on Parks, Protected Areas, and Cultural Sites" (2012), in Samantha Weber, ed., *Rethinking Protected Areas in a Changing World: Proceedings of the 2011 George Wright Society Biennial Conference on Parks, Protected Areas, and Cultural Sites* (Hancock, MI: George Wright Society, 2012).

42. Federal Water Pollution Control Act, 33 U.S.C. §1251 (2002).

43. Ibid., §1251, §101(b). See also *D.C. v. Schramm*, 631 F.2d 854, 860 (D.C. Cir. 1980), which found that "Congress carefully constructed a legislative scheme that imposed major responsibility for control of water pollution on the states." See generally Oliver

A. Houck, "Cooperative Federalism, Nutrients, and the Clean Water Act: Three Cases Revisited," *Environmental Law Institute* 44, no. 5 (2014): 10426.

44. Federal Water Pollution Control Act, 33 U.S.C. §1251, §303.

45. Ibid., §303(e)(3)(a).

46. Ibid., §303.

47. Ibid., §106.

48. Ibid., §105.

49. Ibid., §201–221.

50. See Laura B. Fowler, Matthew B. Royer, and Jamison E. Colburn, "Addressing Death by a Thousand Cuts: Legal and Policy Innovations to Address Nonpoint Source Runoff," Agricultural and Applied Economics Association, *Choices Magazine* (2013), http://choicesmagazine.org/choices-magazine/theme-articles/innovations-in -nonpoint-source-pollution-policy/addressing-death-by-a-thousand-cuts-legal-and -policy-innovations-to-address-nonpoint-source-runoff; and Adena R. Rissman and Stephen R. Carpenter, "Progress on Nonpoint Pollution: Barriers and Opportunities," *Daedalus* 144, no. 3 (2015): 35.

51. See Clean Water Act, 33 U.S.C. §1251, 319 et seq. (1972).

52. See, e.g., "Chesapeake Bay Total Maximum Daily Load (TMDL)," U.S. Environmental Protection Agency, accessed October 9, 2017, https://goo.gl/Vh3jea.

53. Harkinson, "The Landscape-Scarring, Energy-Sucking, Wildlife-Killing Reality of Pot Farming."

54. California Water Boards Media Release, "North Coast Water Board to Hold Workshop May 7 on Marijuana Cultivation," May 4, 2015, http://goo.gl/4ZTh8g.

55. Adrian Fernandez Baumann, "A Carrot and Stick for Pot Farmers," *East Bay Express*, August 12, 2015, http://www.eastbayexpress.com/oakland/a-carrot-and -stick-for-pot-farmers/Content?oid=4454890.

56. One farmer noted that "the water board staff are our preferred regulators because they don't carry guns and badges" (ibid.).

57. Brittany Patterson, "California's 50,000 Pot Farms Are Sucking Rivers Dry," *Scientific American*, July 3, 2015, http://goo.gl/QWdp8H; Tom Huddleston, "The Booming Pot Industry Is Draining the U.S. Energy Supply," *Fortune*, December 21, 2015, http://goo.gl/xWpBfm; Gina S. Warren, "Regulating Pot to Save the Polar Bear: Energy and Climate Impacts of the Marijuana Industry," *Columbia Journal of Environmental Law* 40, no. 3 (2015): 385.

58. Evan Mills, "The Carbon Footprint of Indoor Cannabis Production," *Energy Consumption* 43, no. 35 (2012): 59.

59. Ibid.

60. The 2012 study's findings in Mills's "The Carbon Footprint" have been called into question by some scholars. Given the paucity of information available, what peer-reviewed studies on marijuana agriculture exist must be considered in the context of a rapidly evolving industry.

61. Jennifer Oldham, "As Pot-Growing Expands, Electricity Demands Tax U.S. Grids," *Bloomberg*, December 21, 2015, accessed January 11, 2018, http://goo.gl /JO0dte.

62. One Pennsylvania Public Utility Commissioner said, "We are at the edge of this [...] we are looking all across the country for examples and best practices" (ibid.).

63. Jim Lazar, *Energy Regulation in the U.S.: A Guide*, 8th ed. (Montpelier, VT: Regulatory Assistance Project, 2016), 12.

64. Warren, "Regulating Pot to Save the Polar Bear."

65. Melanie Sevcenko, "Pot Is Power Hungry: Why the Marijuana Industry's Energy Footprint is Growing," *Guardian*, February 27, 2016, http://goo.gl/VI1jU8.

66. Ibid.

67. Medical Marijuana, Boulder, Colorado, Rev. Code §6-14-8(i) (see https:// library.municode.com/co/boulder/codes/municipal_code?nodeId=TIT6HESASA_ CH14MEMA_6-14-8REREOPMEMABU); and Commercial Medical Marijuana Land Use Ordinance, Humboldt County Ordinance No. 2544 (2016).

68. See Res. 2014-41, Board of County Commissioners, Boulder, Colorado (2014), creating the Boulder County Energy Impact Offset Fund.

69. Warren, "Regulating Pot to Save the Polar Bear."

70. Chelsea Harvey, "The Surprisingly Huge Energy Footprint of the Booming Marijuana Industry," *Washington Post*, February 18, 2016, https://goo.gl/SD5BXy.

71. Migoya, "Colorado Yields to Marijuana Industry Pressure on Pesticides."

72. Ibid.

73. According to one survey, 84 percent of Americans purchase organic food, in "U.S. Organic: State of the Industry," Organic Trade Association, 2016, http://goo.gl /RynAkB.

74. Rachael Carson, *Silent Spring* (New York: Houghton Mifflin, 1962).

75. E.g., Clean Water Act, Clean Air Act, Endangered Species Act, National Environmental Protection Act; see also Jedediah Purdy, *After Nature: A Politics for the Anthropocene* (Cambridge, MA: Harvard University Press, 2015).

76. Farming practices prior to the twentieth century are typically considered to have been organic because synthetic pesticides, fertilizers, or genetically modified products had not yet been developed.

77. See Valerie J. Watnick, "The Organic Foods Production Act, the Process/Product Distinction, and a Case for More End Product Regulation in the Organic Foods Market," *UCLA Journal of Environmental Law and Policy* 31, no. 1 (October 2013); Sara N. Pasquinelli, "One False Move: The History of Organic Agriculture and Consequences of Non-Compliance with the Governing Laws and Regulations," *Golden Gate University Environmental Law Journal* 69, no. 2 (Spring 2010): 365.

78. Organic Foods Production Act, 7 U.S.C. §6501 (1990); see also Kyle W. Lathrop, "Pre-Empting Apples with Oranges: Federal Regulation of Organic Food Labeling," *Journal of Corporation Law* 16, no. 4 (June 1991).

79. National Organic Program, 7 U.S.C. §§6501–6522 (1990).

80. Alice Truong, "The Bay Area's Latest Movement: Organic Marijuana," *Quartz*, January 29, 2015, http://goo.gl/WkXYkt.

81. Brian Baker et al., "Organic Farming Compliance Handbook: A Resource Guide for Western Region Agricultural Professionals," University of California Agriculture and Natural Resources, Sustainable Research and Education Program (2005); see also Aubrey Parlet, "Organic Foods Production: What Consumers Might Not Know about the Use of Synthetic Substances," *Loyola Consumer Law Review* 21, no. 3 (2009).

82. Baker et al., "Organic Farming Compliance Handbook."

83. Lathrop, "Pre-Empting Apples with Oranges," 891–892.

84. Ibid.; see also Baker et al., "Organic Farming Compliance Handbook."

85. Compliance Requirement, 7 U.S.C. §6505(a)(1); see also *Quesada v. Herb Thymes Farm Inc.*, 62 Cal. 4th 298 (California 2015).

86. National Organic Production Program, 7 U.S.C. §6503(a).

87. State Organic Certification Program, 7 U.S.C. §6507.

88. But see generally Laura Fisher, "Administrative Law—All (Food) Politics Is Local: Cooperative Federalism, New England Small Farms, and the Food Safety Modernization Act," *Western New England Law Review* 37, no. 3 (2015): 3337. Fisher calls for more state and local involvement in agricultural policy.

89. David Migoya and Ricardo Baca, "Colorado AG's Office Investigates Marijuana Companies Using the Word 'Organic,'" *Denver Post*, August 16, 2015, http://goo.gl /d8tv93. ("'Marijuana may not be certified organic under the USDA organic regulations,' said a USDA spokesman who could not be named because it's the agency's

policy when discussing marijuana. 'Marijuana is considered a controlled substance at the federal level, and organic certification is reserved for agricultural products.'")

90. See e.g., "Clean Green Certified" on the Clean Green Certified website, accessed on October 9, 2017, http://goo.gl/TdZmYU, which explains its origins: "Clean Green Certified was created in 2004 as a way to regulate legal cannabis products that called themselves 'organic.' Consumers can rest assured when they buy a Clean Green cannabis product that it was tested and found free of synthetic pesticides, fungicides, moldicides. Modeled on national and international organic and sustainability standards, the Clean Green program requires on-site inspections and third-party lab testing. Much like the USDA National Organic Program for traditional agricultural products, the whole life cycle of the plant is considered, from seed selection to harvesting and processing, as well as soil, nutrients, pesticide use, mold treatment and dust control." See also "How Sustainable Do You Want to Be?," Certified Kind, accessed on January 13, 2018, http://goo.gl/q0ZFU9, which explains: "Since USDA Organic certification is not yet allowed for cannabis, Certified Kind exists to offer certification for the organic cannabis farmer and processor. Certified Kind growers are able to use the Certified Kind name and logo to differentiate their crop and support earth-friendly cannabis production."

91. Truong, "The Bay Area's Latest Movement."

92. "Organic," Colorado Department of Agriculture, accessed March 29, 2016, https://goo.gl/s4o7JD.

93. Migoya and Baca, "Colorado AG's Office Investigates Marijuana Companies Using the Word 'Organic.'"

94. This could occur for reasons similar to the benefits of appellations. See Rachael E. Goodhue et al., "California Wine Industry Evolving to Compete in 21st Century," *California Agriculture* 62, no. 1 (2008): 16–17.

95. Erik Chavez et al., "An End-to-End Assessment of Extreme Weather Impacts on Food Security," *Natural Climate Change* 5 (2015): 997. Chavez et al. write: "changes in the large-scale climate processes that drive both regional and global climate variability affect the annual onset of rainfall in the tropics and subtropics, as well as rainfall patterns in temperate latitudes, thus playing a significant role in the variability of regional rain-fed crop production." See also Mark R. Rosenzweig and Hans P. Binswanger, "Wealth, Weather and the Composition and Profitability of Agricultural Investment," *Economic Journal* 103, no. 416 (1993): 56.

96. Steffen N. Johnson, "A Regulatory 'Wasteland': Defining a Justified Federal Role in Crop Insurance," *North Dakota Law Review* 72 (1996): 507, citing 126 Congressional Record 2,737 (1980) (statement of Rep. Ed Jones).

97. See J. Beddington et al., *Achieving Food Security in the Face of Climate Change: Final Report from the Commission on Sustainable Agriculture and Climate Change*, CGIAR Research Program on Climate Change (2012).

98. Ralph M. Chite, "Emergency Funding for Agriculture: A Brief History of Supplemental Appropriations, FY1989–FY2009," Congressional Research Service (2012).

99. Ibid.

100. Erwann Michel-Kerjan and Jacquelin Volkman-Wise, "The Risk of Ever-Growing Disaster Relief Expectations," Risk Management and Decision Process Center, Wharton School of the University of Pennsylvania, 2011.

101. Darrell L. Hueth and William F. Furtan, eds., *Economics of Agriculture Crop Insurance: Theory and Evidence* (New York: Kluwer Academic Publishers, 1994).

102. Michel-Kerjan and Volkman-Wise, "The Risk of Ever-Growing Disaster Relief Expectations," 3.

103. Federal Crop Insurance Act 7 U.S.C. §1505 (1938).

104. Johnson, "A Regulatory 'Wasteland,'" 507, citing H.R. 649, 103d Congress, Second Session, 20 (1994).

105. See Agricultural Act of 2014, Public Law 113-79 (2014).

106. Dennis A. Shields, "Federal Crop Insurance: Background," Congressional Research Service, August 13, 2015, https://fas.org/sgp/crs/misc/R40532.pdf.

107. Ibid., 2.

108. In 2012, costs peaked at $14.1 billion; in 2014, costs declined to $8.7 billion (ibid.).

109. See "County Crop Programs," USDA Risk Management Agency, United States Department of Agriculture, accessed October 9, 2017, http://goo.gl/2z6GIi.

110. See, e.g., Ed Leefeldt, "For Insurers, No Rush to Offer Pot Coverage," *CBS Money Watch*, February 24, 2016, http://goo.gl/HdGQfQ.

111. See, e.g., Paul Rogers, "California Drought: How Will We Know When It's Over?," *San Jose Mercury News*, January 9, 2016, http://goo.gl/54dQlx.

112. See Madeleine Thomas, "West Coast Weed Farms Are Lighting Up: As Wildfires Continue to Ravage the West Coast, Concerns Emerge for the Marijuana Industry," *Pacific Standard*, August 31, 2015, http://goo.gl/CrpQMl.

113. See, e.g., Michael Roberts, "Medical Marijuana Crop Insurance: Putting Your Weed in Good Hands," *Westword*, February 10, 2010, http://goo.gl/V1J6B2. Roberts's 2010 article shows that early crop insurance policies covered only indoor growing operations.

114. *Tracy v. USAA Casualty Ins. Co.*, no. 11-00487 WL 928186 (D. Haw. 2012).

115. Ibid., 25.

116. Ibid., 32.

117. *Green Earth Wellness Center LLC. v. Atain Specialty Insurance Co.*, No.-13-03452-MSK-NYW WL 632357 (D. Colo. 2016).

118. Ibid., 22.

119. One could argue that a price collapse would have positive public health impacts by making those marijuana strains with medicinal and therapeutic benefits more accessible to low-income consumers.

Chapter 9

1. https://www.monticello.org/site/plantation-and-slavery/hem.

2. The Senate had never before used the nuclear option to end debate on a Supreme Court nominee. Senate Democrats, however, were the first to invoke the nuclear option at all when they used it to end debate on President Obama's nominees for other judicial and executive branch appointments in 2013.

3. Nick Visser, "Sen. Jeff Merkley Stages All-Night Protest on Senate Floor against Gorsuch Nomination," Politics, *Huffington Post*, April 5, 2017, https://www.huffingtonpost.com/entry/jeff-merkley-senate-protest_us_58e466f8e4b03a26a367750d.

4. Ibid.

5. A Resolution Designating the Week of June 5 Through June 11, 2017, as "Hemp History Week," S. Res. 189, 115th Congress (2017), https://www.congress.gov/bill/115th-congress/senate-resolution/189/text.

6. "Bipartisan Coalition of Senators Designates Hemp History Week: Resolution by Wyden, McConnell, Merkley and Paul Recognizes Economic Potential for Industrial Hemp Farming in the United States," Ron Wyden: Senator for Oregon, June 9, 2017, accessed October 11, 2017, https://www.wyden.senate.gov/news/press-releases/bipartisan-coalition-of-senators-designates-hemp-history-week-.

7. Kentucky's Agriculture Commissioner stated in 2015 that "hemp equals jobs and true economic growth." The same year, one of the state's U.S. Representatives said, "For far too long, farmers and manufacturers in Kentucky and across the United States have been blocked from growing hemp or producing products from this versatile and useful plant. My colleagues and I in both the House and Senate hope to end this illogical ban."

8. Oregon's other U.S. Senator, Ron Wyden, called the federal cannabis prohibition an "unjustifiable ban on growing hemp … locking American farmers and innovators out of good-paying jobs and countless ways to profit from this versatile plant." See "Bipartisan Coalition of Senators Designates Hemp History Week."

9. A Resolution Designating the Week of June 5 Through June 11, 2017, as "Hemp History Week."

10. Renee Johnson, "Hemp as an Agricultural Commodity," Congressional Research Service, RL32725 (Washington D.C.: CRS, March 2017), accessed October 11, 2017, https://fas.org/sgp/crs/misc/RL32725.pdf

11. Industrial Hemp Farming Act of 2015, S. 134, 114th Congress (2015).

12. See Renee Johnson, "Vote Hemp: 2016 Hemp Update," Congressional Update, Congressional Research Service, RL32725 (Washington, D.C.: CRS, 2016), accessed April 9, 2018, http://goo.gl/Y2K77S.

13. Johnson, "Hemp as an Agricultural Commodity."

14. Martin Booth, *Cannabis: A History* (New York: St. Martin's Press, 2005).

15. Jack Herer, *The Emperor Wears No Clothes*, 12th ed. (Van Nuys, CA: Ah Ha Publishing, 2011), originally published in 1985.

16. Johnson, "Hemp as an Agricultural Commodity."

17. Timing is important: too much decomposition ruins the fibers, whereas too little decomposition won't provide access to the fibers.

18. Doug Fine, *Hemp Bound: Dispatches from the Front Lines of the Next Agricultural Revolution* (White River Junction, VT: Chelsea Green Publishing, 2014), 10.

19. Ibid., 17.

20. Herer, *The Emperor Wears No Clothes*, 87.

21. Fine, *Hemp Bound*, 13.

22. Johnson, "Hemp as an Agricultural Commodity."

23. See Fine, *Hemp Bound*, 67.

24. Ibid., 25.

25. Alexa Peduzzi, "The Hipster's Smoothie," *Fooduzzi* (blog), accessed October 11, 2017, https://www.fooduzzi.com/2015/01/the-hipsters-smoothie/.

26. Quoted in Fine, *Hemp Bound*, 128.

27. Ibid., 99–100.

28. See Koichi Sakamoto et al., "Characterization: Genome Sizes and Morphology of Sex Chromosomes in Hemp (Cannabis sativa L.)," *Cytologia* 63, no. 4 (1998): 459.

29. See "Identifying Cannabis Plants Gender," Cannabis Cure, accessed April 9, 2018, https://www.cannabiscure.info/cannabis-plant-gender/.

30. In some cases, pollination has been observed across a thirty-mile distance. See Knut Faegri and Johs Iversen, *Textbook of Pollen Analysis*, 6th ed. (Caldwell, NJ: Blackburn Press, 2000); Baltasar Cabezudo et al., "Atmospheric Transportation of Marihuana Pollen from North Africa to the Southwest of Europe," *Atmospheric Environment* 31, no. 20 (1997): 3323; Sofia Kutuzova et al., "Maintenance of Cannabis Germplasm in the Vavilov Research Institute Gene Bank," *Journal of the International Hemp Association* 4, no. 1 (1996): 17–18; Ernest Small and Tanya Antle, "A Preliminary Study of Pollen Dispersal in *Cannabis sativa* in Relation to Wind Direction," *Journal of Industrial Hemp* 8, no. 2 (2003): 44; Joy Beckerman, "Myths of Cannabis and Hemp Cross-Pollination: Myths and Realities of Cross-Pollination," *Seattle Pi* (blog), April 8, 2015, http://goo.gl/hl7xtD.

31. Many states mirror the 0.3 percent THC content requirement found in the Industrial Hemp Farming Act of 2015, including Connecticut, Minnesota, Montana, and New Hampshire; see An Act Legalizing Industrial Hemp, Conn. Pub. Acts 15-202 (2015); Industrial Hemp Development, Minn. Stat. §§18k.01–18k.04; Industrial Hemp, Mont. Code Ann. §80-18-101; Industrial Hemp Defined, N.H. Rev. Stat. Ann. §433-C:1 (2015).

32. Agricultural Act of 2014, Public Law 113-79, §7606, 113th Congress (2014).

33. See Keith Mansur, "Cannabis Appellation Regions for Oregon: A Solution for Unwanted Cross-Pollination of Hemp and Marijuana," *Oregon Cannabis Connection*, July 22, 2016, accessed January 12, 2018, https://olis.leg.state.or.us/liz/2015R1/Downloads/CommitteeMeetingDocument/78941.

34. See Detlef Bartsch et al., "Environmental Implications of Gene Flow from Sugar Beet to Wild Beet—Current Status and Future Research Needs," *Environmental Biosafety Research* 2, no. 2 (2003): 105; Kent Brittan, "Methods to Enable Coexistence of Diverse Corn Production Systems," *Agricultural Biotechnology in California Series* 8192 (2006): 1.

35. For a discussion of the European Union's extensive crop coexistence regulations, see Koreen Ramessar et al., "Going to Ridiculous Lengths—European Coexistence Regulations for GM Crops," *Nature Biotechnology* 28, no. 133 (2010): 133, doi:10.1038/nbt0210-133.

36. This is common in corn cultivation. See ibid., and Brittan, "Methods to Enable Coexistence of Diverse Corn Production Systems," 3.

37. Industrial Hemp Research Program, Washington Administrative Code, 16-305 (2017), http://apps.leg.wa.gov/wac/default.aspx?cite=16-305&full=true.

38. Again, this is a commonly proposed technique for corn cultivation. See Brittan, "Methods to Enable Coexistence of Diverse Corn Production Systems," 4.

39. Covering plants to prevent cross-fertilization is more popular for small-scale gardening. As discussed in chapter 7, indoor agriculture's energy footprint is extensive,

particularly with respect to indoor marijuana; see Evan Mills, "Energy up in Smoke: The Carbon Footprint of Indoor Cannabis Production," *Energy Policy* 46 (2012): 58; and Jennifer Oldham, "As Pot-Growing Expands, Electricity Demands Tax U.S. Grids," *Bloomberg*, December 21, 2015, accessed January 11, 2018, http://goo.gl /JO0dte.

40. See Mansur, "Cannabis Appellation Regions for Oregon," 5–6.

41. See Fine, *Hemp Bound*.

42. See Mansur, "Cannabis Appellation Regions for Oregon," 7. Mansur argues that "Oregon should adopt a cannabis appellation system to help prevent problems likely to arise from cultivation of differing industrial hemp varieties low in THC and the high THC varieties of marijuana needed for the medical and adult use markets" (7).

43. Matthew Korfhage, "Why Hemp and Marijuana Farmers Had a Messy Breakup—and What Happens Now," *Potlander* (blog), *Willamette Week*, November 8, 2016, http://www.wweek.com/cannabis/2016/10/04/why-hemp-and-marijuana-farmers -had-a-messy-breakup-and-what-happens-now/.

Chapter 10

1. William Howard Taft, "Address Accepting the Republican Presidential Nomination," The American Presidency Project, accessed on October 17, 2017, http://www .presidency.ucsb.edu/ws/index.php?pid=76222.

2. "American Presidents on the Importance of Agriculture," Farm Policy Facts (website), accessed October 17, 2017, https://www.farmpolicyfacts.org/2016/02/american -presidents-on-the-importance-of-agriculture/.

3. Cathleen D. Cahill, *Federal Fathers and Mothers: A Social History of the United States Indian Service, 1869–1933* (Chapel Hill: University of North Carolina Press, 2011), 309.

4. The fact that white federal officials favored agriculture over subsistence hunting and gathering no doubt played a role in their decision as well.

5. David R. Lewis, *Neither Wolf nor Dog: American Indians, Environment, and Agrarian Change* (Oxford: Oxford University Press, 1994), 98.

6. Ibid., 100.

7. Ibid., 105.

8. Ibid.

9. Will Houston, "Hoopa Tribe Set to Make Emergency Declaration Due to Crime," *Eureka Times-Standard*, February 17, 2016, http://www.times-standard.com/article/NJ /20160217/NEWS/160219875.

10. Wendell Berry, *The Unsettling of America: Culture and Agriculture* (1977; repr., Berkeley, CA: Counterpoint Press, 2015), 44.

11. Ibid., 45–46.

12. Ibid., 47.

13. Michael Carolan has written thoughtfully about the long-term costs of low-priced agricultural products. See, generally, Michael S. Carolan, *Reclaiming Food Security* (New York: Routledge Press, 2013).

14. Berry, *The Unsettling of America*, 51.

15. Ibid., 62.

Index